Beautiful Dreamer

Pamela Pickton

All rights reserved, no part of this publication may be reproduced by any means, electronic, mechanical photocopying, documentary, film or in any other format without prior written permission of the publisher.

Published by
Chipmunkapublishing
PO Box 6872
Brentwood
Essex CM13 1ZT
United Kingdom

http://www.chipmunkapublishing.com

Copyright © 2012

Front cover: author's mother
Eleanor Matthews **née** Rainer
daughter of Mildred Rainer **née** Peircey
daughter of George Peircey, of the Percy line

Chipmunkapublishing gratefully acknowledges the support of Arts Council England.

Pamela Pickton

Dedicated to my eldest daughter
KAREN DUNN
A first girl like Nan and me.

Beautiful Dreamer

Pamela Pickton

'Suffocated by longing,
her poor old heart gave
out.'

(Source unknown)

Beautiful Dreamer

The Song Of The Little Match Girl

Sometimes I die of hunger. Other times I freeze to death.

Another time I come in the form of Cinderella: I
sweep and drudge with no prospect of the pretty
dress, the handsome Prince.

Or you might find me dressed as Snow White,
whom older, bitter people seek to destroy.

You could see me locked up in some kind of
fortress, too far away from an exit to ever hope of escape.

There, I am married to a Blue Beard, who will never
allow me into the secret chamber of his heart,
because he has lost the key himself.

And here I am living with a Beast who, like all
beasts, is a Prince in disguise, but who cannot set
free his real self.

In many forms I come, a Sleeping Beauty,
waiting and waiting until my breath runs out.

Written by Pamela Pickton after being inspired by
the first line. (Author unknown)

Beautiful Dreamer

Chapter 1

'….And she's got a perfect figure, you know.' For the first time I am listening to what the nurse is saying about my eighty-eight year-old mother.

'I like her,' she had begun. What's all this? I asked myself. My mother's never got on with anybody, and probably nobody has ever liked her. She certainly doesn't like anyone much. The nurse carries on talking as I scrabble around, trying to remember how the conversation had started. 'She asks me where I came from. Tells me she has always wanted to travel…' Well, we all know that old story, don't we?

'…And she's got a perfect figure, you know.' That's when my ears pricked up. I'd hardly been listening, having looked after my mother for as long as I can remember, having lived her life rather than my own… But now this, at nearly ninety and last week nearly dead. 'What do you mean, what do you mean? In and out –in and out?'

'Oh – everything,' the nurse laughs. 'And it is good for you, because it's genetic.' Genetic? I am her, not exactly a case of symbiosis, since it has not been beneficial to me, but something like that.

A week ago, I stood over my mother, having been
summoned to what I had thought was her deathbed. She was asleep, but gasping in her sleep, and I thought, 'Are you gasping to stay alive in the hope that one day you will have a life?' No, what I really thought was, you look like I feel. Gasping to stay alive in the hope that one day I will have a life. And now this, the perfect figure? A young girl's body beneath that weary face? The tune `Beautiful Dreamer` comes into my mind. I think she even used to sing it, way far back, or at least hum it anyway, a Sleeping Beauty, is it really that? Is that old face weary with disappointment? Because the young
girl's body has never been satisfied? Yet my mother has never shown any strong desires for such needs to be fulfilled. I am a Sleeping Beauty too, but I know it.

All I can remember of my mother is that she was always scruffy, almost dirty, and in hindsight I realise she was probably no role model of how to be feminine. No eyelash fluttering, no pouting and I can remember no innocent flirting with any man in our life. Widowed at barely sixty, there was never any sign of her wanting to marry again, or even taking a lover. She went to a club for widowed people in those days, and once she told me that a man had walked her to the bus stop.

'Oh,' I responded. 'Would you... I mean, would you ever...?'

The next day she called me with all the usual vitriol. 'What you said yesterday, about me marrying again. You only want me to, so that you don't have to do it.'

Do what? Be her husband? I Some of us even thought that my mother may have had lesbian tendencies. However, what I do remember is that she rejected a lot of programmes on television because there was too much of 'that nasty business.' Once, she and my father went to see a Marriage Guidance Counsellor, but she gave up on them ever being able to help her. '...because they just go on about sex,' she spat at me.

On the other hand, when overtly asked by her young,
married daughters, she had said that she had not liked 'all of that' because, 'he was not nice to all of you.'

The guilt at my mother's misery had been set in motion
early. 'Soon be in my box and never seen the world.' I
caught and held those words, a small child of three. When I asked her how old she was, she said ninety-nine. I knew she was thirty years older than me so I must have been good at sums already as I worked out she was thirty three. She had 'one foot in the grave,' she kept saying, and I remember now my feeling of horror and even of physical sickness. And so my life`s mission was set in progress.

(Were these the days of the tea? Mother has told me that, when I was very small, if ever asked to carry a cup of tea to her, I did it so slowly, so carefully. So successfully. Already bearing gifts to my mother. Or trying to. A cup of tea carried beseechingly on a saucer, like a golden chalice on a cushion of silk.)

Then, when I was six, my mother was ill in hospital. I did not know what was wrong with her at the time, but I found out later that she had had a miscarriage. I missed my mum. I was worried about my mum, and I needed attention from somebody. I was alone with my dad one evening when my sister, much younger, was in bed and my older brother, who listened to the radio a lot, was in another room because it was time for 'Dick Barton.'

I asked my dad to comb out my hair, because it was
tangled, so that it would look better the next day for school. But I was a nuisance. He had two other children to look after, and could not spend time on my hair. 'If Mum dies, it will be your fault,' he told me. So it was instilled in me from a young age, and I believed it for most of my life, that my mother's unhappiness was my fault, and that I had to do something about it. I worked hard at school and aimed at University and
a good job, so that I could take my mother round the world.

Now fresh images flicker back and forth like slides in the memory being thrown on my screen as I look at my mother anew, and wonder if I have been getting it wrong all my life. I had always thought it was money she wanted, and travel of course.

She had collapsed, and nearly died, whilst 'out and about.' She had been found by a stranger near a riverside seat in Surbiton, and taken by ambulance to hospital where, the doctors told us, they had spent two hours bringing her back to life. What could have been her last moments were out in the fresh air, amidst green places and by the river she loved. Did she feel ill before she left home, yet somehow dragged herself to what was more her home?

Yes, going out, and the money to go further, did seem to be, for her, what to most women might be like running for President of the Parent's Association, getting involved with a political party, having an affair if married, or going to the Singles Club if not.

She sent off her football coupons like someone else sends off their novels, or at least writes letters to the
newspapers – looking for something which might bring recognition, fulfillment, or at least a chance.

Mother did in fact have a letter published in a national
newspaper once. It was saying how being married to the Manager of a Newsagent's Shop was a hard life, but instead of praise she got attack. Her family were angry at her complaining

about a way of life which more than one of them had, and the wife of a milkman wrote to her saying she should count her blessings for her lot was far worse.

Someone who ran a newspaper shop in those days got up at four in the morning to get the papers out. Presumably it is the same now. So then they have the aggravation of paper boys not turning up, irate customers on the telephone complaining, and maybe having to take the newspapers out themselves usually, in those days, on a bicycle. If the family lived behind the shop, then they would have the staff using their bathroom, and have to provide them with refreshments.

Certainly, at that time, the Manager of a Newsagents shop was one of the poorest paid workers in the country. In my early childhood, we lived in a small rented flat which was shabby, both in decoration and furnishings. The shiny green paint used to blister and burst showing the plaster beneath, and we had coats on the beds as blankets. Our clothes were a constant source of embarrassment. In post war England many people were poor, but I knew that my clothes were the
worst in the school, and this poverty lasted all the time I lived at home. At the age of ten, I had to wear the dress of an elderly neighbour. It had a rosette on the bodice, which was made out of the same material as the dress. I hated wearing an old-lady dress.

I shudder now at the embarrassment when a well-to-do
visitor was asked if he would like a cup of tea, and replied that he only wanted a glass of water. I knew he said this in order to save us the cost of tea, milk and the electricity to boil the water, but it was equally as devastating for us because we did not own any drinking glasses.

My father had never planned on working in a shop. When, at the age of eleven, I found my parents' Marriage Certificate, his occupation was stated as that of a 'Piano Tuner'. He had left school at a very early age, and for the second half of his childhood had been an orphan. However, he was clearly talented, being an able businessman, quick at adding up money whilst running the shop, and playing the piano by ear. In the army he had played the trombone in an orchestra, and
in my childhood, as well as working in the shop, he made and decorated wedding cakes for extra money. At another stage in

our lives, he was employed on his afternoon off by another shop, as a window dresser.

After the war, he wanted to train as a chiropodist. However we lived in the same London district where 'the shop' was situated, the shop owned by my grandmother, and run by my mother's brother. The family persuaded him to go and work for them, and I have often wondered why we were so poor. If he were family, why did they not pay him over the odds and give us a more decent wage? Why not give him shares in the business, and for life, even when he moved away and managed another shop for low wages?

The long hours in the shop would have made life hard for my mother anyway, but on top of that my father was persuaded to sleep there, so not coming home to his wife and children, except on Sunday, although the shop was only streets away. And so my mother was locked up alone with domesticity, poverty, and children. She felt the walls closing in on her, the ceiling pressing down on her head. What she liked was fresh air, open green spaces, and what she called 'nice places.'

She also liked a café where she could have a cup of tea which she had not made herself. But even that was not enough, what she wanted most of all in life was to travel. 'I want to be free,' she would say. 'I would like to be a gypsy, never in the same place long, constantly moving on, going from place to place, out in the fresh air.' There was a song around at the time, it seemed to be her theme song – 'Don't Fence Me In.'

Sadly, there was no gypsy caravan, and of course no car in our family until the last decade of my father's life. I recall how, when there was a General Election, my mother would vote for any party whose members came and picked her up in a car to go to the Polling Station!

'Gertcha, gertcha,' Mother would curse at the cars that prevented us from crossing the road, when she had a pram and a gaggle of children in tow. 'I curse you, I curse...' Did she curse because they were in our way, or because those people had cars?

She even envied dogs in cars. In fact she hated to see a dog being, as it seemed to her, given a ride in a car. Never mind dogs probably dislike going in cars. To her they were being given nice outings, and more than she ever got.

Gypsies. Travel. Cars. Those I thought all my life were
the stuff my mother's dreams were made of, the lack of which resulted in all her ills. Now, as I drive home from the hospital, the nurse's words about a 'perfect figure' and the idea those words echo. bringing thoughts of my mother as a Sleeping Beauty, make me wonder if I have been getting it wrong.

A scene, lost for thirty years, flashes before me. It
happened a few weeks before my sister's wedding. Valerie, who was still living at home, was doing her hand washing in the kitchen sink, and leaving puddles of water all over the floor. Now, Mother could stand nor sight nor sound of housework. Whether it nudged her of her own neglect in that area, or she just did not want to be reminded that such chores existed, I do not know.

All I do know is that she does not want to be discomfited, and the puddles on the floor would have been an irritation, if not an 'eyesore', and they might mean she had to mop the floor after the clothes had been washed. Mother always made a big 'to-do' about her weekly cleaning of that floor and everybody had to go out and buy fish and chips rather than make more work for her.

Mother screeched at my sister, and my sister screeched back that she, a bride in two week's time, should not have to be doing her own washing. The screeching turned into a fight, the kind of a struggle that I had seen before, sometimes between my father and sister, and then my mother scratched her own daughter's face. Although the scratches were healed in time for the wedding, they were deep enough to need medical attention. I thought, all those years ago, that envy was behind the attack, the envy of a new start, of a husband with a better job, a husband with a car.

I had always believed that my mother's misery was due to that – lack of a car, travel, and the basic lack of money to provide those things. Surely that was the reasoning behind the frantic doing of the pools, so religiously, every week? She never missed a week, not even on family holidays where she did them sitting on a deckchair on the stony beach at Southend, or huddled up on the windy pier.

All my life I have been so immersed in my mother's misery, trying to make things better for her. To understand is part of he way to healing I have always thought, but the conversation with the nurse in my mother's present hospital has started me on a different tack in that understanding. Could that animal like scratching of my sister's face have come from some deep jealousy that my sister was about to have a sexual chance? But Mother had never liked sex, had
she? What about 'that nasty business'? What about my
father? She had a husband after all.

What comes back to me now is the picture of my mother and how she was when she talked to us. She was never still, her hands going all over her body, tracing her outlines, her contours. In particular she would rub her hands over the roundness of her breasts and bottom, always rubbing herself, touching her hair, and turning her head from side to side. I had always seen this as part of her general restlessness, but now it is as if I am seeing things with a different lens, a different filter.

As I lock the car and go into my house a sort of heaviness comes over me, a lifetime's knowledge of Mother's incessant visits to doctors and clinics, sometimes hospitals. Always unwell, always troubled. Forever going somewhere with unclear complaints, and coming back unsatisfied, or with a bottle of 'tonic'. For a short time the National Health Service offered a service to women of retirement age, a clinic which was held monthly, where you were given advice on diet and
lifestyle, and a thorough physical examination. 'It is good at that clinic,' I remember her telling me. 'They go all over you.'

Was the 'going-all-over' merely a reassurance of physical safety, or did she actually enjoy it in itself? My new perspective is making me rethink this now. As I have mentioned, my sister and I had wondered at the possibility of a lesbian tendency, and that could certainly explain the desire for touch when she made it fairly clear that she did not like sex. Of course, the claim of disliking the act could have been due to what sex had meant to her. There was the pain of childbirth and the drudgery brought upon her by raising four children with little money. Would sex have been different for her had she been comfortably off? Would she have desired a man who could take her out and about in a car? Or better still, a camper van? For once those vehicles appeared on the roads, they had gradually replaced the gypsy caravan of her dreams.

I had always tried to understand my mother, and now that I have a new lead, old memories come back as though I have awoken a part of my brain where there has been stored a dusty collection of old transparencies. The scenes are always the same, of Mother standing there stroking herself. And I realise I often find myself doing it too.

The old clinic's nurses 'went all over her,' and she 'went all over' herself. There was, it seems, a definite need to be touched, but was that the baby's need for cuddles and strokes – which, it is highly likely, were thin on the ground for her – or was it some need of her adult self? If the latter, why was it not satisfied within her marriage? Was it because of her poverty, or was it something else, something much deeper? Maybe she just did not realise that she was stroking herself, or did not even know why she was doing it. Can one be unaware of sexual needs, especially if there are other problems clouding it? 'A Sleeping Beauty,' I had thought to myself when the nurse first told me of the young girl's body beneath the aging face. Why does the face show so much age? Is it because it is in the mind behind the eyes that the pain is registered, as hope fades and dies? 'A Sleeping Beauty' who has waited nearly ninety years for a Prince who has never come? Or has my mother in fact been Snow White, keeping herself in a perpetual glass case?

Of course to wake from that suspended animation, which was Snow White's brief state and Sleeping Beauty's hundred year one, would bring adulthood with its possibility of fulfillment – yes – but also that other possibility of disappointment. And to become adult is also to begin on what is, after all, the journey downhill, to old age and to death.

My mother does afford some smiles as well though. When she was going to the loved clinic for the over sixties (and I was in my thirties) she was always telling that I could look forward to going there one day. As if I would wish half my life away for that nice little outing.

Chapter 2

Another hospital visit and I arrive in time to catch Mother spitting out pills. There is no nurse by the bed now, so she must have kept them in the corner of her mouth until safely alone. What is even more amazing is that the tongue is pushing out the pills even though she is almost asleep. I can't talk to her, she is dozy and her eyes are closed.

'I won't stay for long, Mother,' I say. I sit by the bed awhile, wondering at the fighting spirit, spitting out pills whilst gasping to stay alive.

I have always thought of my mother as downtrodden, and suppressed, certainly not living a life of her choice. On the one hand she seemed to take it – albeit nagging all the time – like the times I witnessed my father bashing her on the back. There was very often a look on her face of some kind of submission. Her facial expression was commonly apologetic, pleading, sometime guilt ridden. She would often talk with her hand over her mouth.

Once, when I was seeing her off after a day with me, I left her to walk the last few yards to the bus stop alone, so that I could get back to my children. She fell and scurried back to me, her hand over her mouth again, blood on her face. The look was one of 'I am a terrible person. This is my fault, I am in trouble again. It is my fault and all that I deserve. it is my fault for falling over.'

Perhaps I read all that into her expression because I know that is how I look and feel sometimes. Now I wonder if it came from the time she told me that, in her babyhood, her mother broke her arm, an accident which Mother believed she had caused.

The whole body language of expecting no less, a kind of defeat, was all over her as my father thumped her on the back. And yet at the same time, alongside all of that, there has always been that rebellion, that fighting spirit, like spitting out her pills today.

Defeat and rebellion, acceptance and protest, these sum my mother up. One of the ways this duality would manifest was in her whole attitude to being given presents. With birthdays, Christmas, and Mother's Day, it was all too often, 'I don't want any presents, don't give me any presents.' In the case of

Mother's Day, right up to now, it has been, 'I don't deserve any presents. I have not been a good mother.' Then, after we had done our best, without any idea of what to give her, and usually with little money, it would be, 'what I really wanted was...'

But her true spirit, the real wants, amidst all the 'don't wants' and the 'don't deserves,' burst through when she wrote us a list. For amongst the combs, hankies, bath salts, scarves and face creams, were slipped in between, the 'Coach Tour' and the 'World Cruise.' 'I don't deserve,' yet at the same time her real self owned its desired delights – and in pushing its head out through her mask of lowliness, perhaps bleated some slight belief of deserving?

She was never pleased by any gift, and I have long wondered if she would have been if it had been the coach tour or the world cruise. My father did later provide her with coach trips, when his shop became an agency for a coach business, and she did enjoy those. Usually, however good the presents, the combs and things from her list or even something a bit special from Dad, like a blouse, she could never show any gratitude. From a young age I came to the conclusion that she did not want us to think that she was all right, that the present had not improved anything for her, or made her happier.

For many years she begged for a gold chain to wear around her neck. When we finally clubbed together to buy her one, she undid the parcel, crumpled up the paper and threw that on the floor, then said it was not the kind she wanted. She rarely wore it, and broke it soon after.

I look at her lying in the bed, eyes closed.

'Don't think I'm all right now,' I always believed she was saying. I didn't think beyond that, but now I see that there may have been a pain which nothing, certainly no present, could assuage – except its healing.

I suppose the biggest rebellion has always been the going out, the refusal to stay at home so that she could do the housework and produce clean and mended clothes for her children. She wanted to get out of the house as much as she could, whether to the shops or cafés or to jumble sales. This behaviour was condemned by her relatives and viewed as 'gallivanting, gadding about and frittering,' because of course it meant less time for housework, and less money too. Now, with my new lens, I see it all as part of a brave, defiant, and determined spirit which was providing her with some palliative at least, if not cure.

She took us with her of course, and I wonder if the constant being out caused the agoraphobia which I have suffered all my adult life. I felt lost and bleak in the countryside or in wild parks, and the trees and skies did not offer me the solace they offered to most, and obviously to her. They were alien, frightening, and I longed to be home.

Once, when we were in the street market of a different town, I had come adrift from the family. I remember wondering if I would ever sleep in my bed that night. I do believe that she thought she was doing her best for us, getting us out of our limiting home environment and showing us a much wider horizon. She bought us sweets and ice-creams, ice lollies and comics. Of course, she was giving us what she thought everyone must love as much as her, the great outdoors. When she no longer had children under school age at home, she could go further, and was off on buses to more distant towns or on coaches to the seaside.

The second half of her life has been spent in the Thames Valley and she loved the river, enjoying sitting by it, and by trees. One of her newer ventures was to visit the Spiritualist Church, where she had been told that to sit near trees and water is healing.

She always told us children that if ever she won the pools she was going to send us all to Boarding School. I always wondered why, as we were not troublesome children. Of course I knew her main dream of winning the pools would have been the travel, with a camper van in the shape of a car. Getting away, getting rid of, or running away from responsibility, that was her ambition. But if her dreams were never realised beyond the gallivanting and gadding about, there was still that air of rebellion and protest in those aims.

There was a kind of rebellion in the way she stood alone. She was not going to be put into any box, not labelled as a housewife, certainly not as `common` or `ordinary`, which is why she joined no women's groups. To this day she rejects, and objects, to the singing of 'Daisy Daisy' because she sees it as the world putting a certain generation into some entertainment box.

More than once she did try to run away from her family, but it was probably hardly recognised, especially as we would have been at school and she was so often out anyway. She would get as far as one of the big London terminuses and then telephone my father. It was always the same, she would explain that she was running away and he would persuade her to come back home, the main intention behind making the call, I think. Otherwise why make it, why not just go? But where would she have gone, and how would she have managed? She had no income, no money.

She was always running, or wishing to run, from domesticity and the tie of children. But was that so rare? Was it unforgivable? Today things are so different, the young mothers with their gym memberships, lunch parties and further education opportunities – not to mention crèches, nursery schools, nannies and au pairs – have a different way of life. I see a large majority of them not having to undergo the privation of the post war bride. They have spare money and aren't accused of gallivanting or frittering when they want to go out. As for foreign travel, we take that for granted, and nowadays almost everyone has had some taste of it.

The brave adventurous spirit was always there. Once, there was a bus strike in her area, which meant that she couldn't get to Hampton Court Palace or Kew Gardens. The only bus running was going to New Malden, which boasted neither park nor river. It was all that was available, so she went. Given her limitations, how less pioneering was that than putting a rucksack on her back and walking round the world?

Running away Is what people called her endless going out. Running away from responsibility, but maybe she was running away from herself, too? Or was it from her suffering? No one ever stopped to consider that, including me. Defeat and acceptance balanced by rebellion and protest, acted out by actually running, or dreaming of greater running. It has always been obvious to me that my mother would want to run from poverty and ties, but now I wonder if there was some greater demon from which she could never escape, because it was inside her.

Maybe there has been a definite childishness about her method of rebelling? Her rejecting children's little gifts, of running and not running away. Perhaps if more adult and more developed, she might have found a better life. She could have got out of her marriage, found herself employment, have nurtured something in herself which might have made her life more enjoyable, her pain more bearable.

What stunted that emotional growth? The words the nurse said to me made me want to examine my mother in depth, for she has always been childish, and I have simply accepted it, until now. Spitting out the pills like a naughty child who is not going to do as 'Mummy' says is good for it.

She has fallen asleep as I've been watching her, her tongue moving the pills to the edge of her mouth. Now they have sunk back, and I am telling myself that they must have dissolved, must have gone down her throat. What else can I tell myself? No nurse is nearby, and I do not know what to do.

*

A week later, and I am walking into the hospital again, this time with my youngest daughter Imogen, who has come up from Wiltshire to visit her grandmother. She is a teacher, it is the school holidays, and she is always glad of an opportunity to stay with me, see her siblings and catch up with old school friends. Imogen is the only one of my four children who lives at a distance, but we both write to each other every week and speak on the telephone twice weekly.

We walk past beds where old people lie with mouths open, sleeping, dozing, pretending to be asleep, or perhaps dead. We can see Mother, at the end of the ward, and she is definitely not dead. She is sitting propped up on the bed, and has other visitors – one of her nephews and her only niece. I am not sure that I would know who they are if my cousin Elaine had not called me on hearing of my mother's collapse, and told me she would ask one of her brothers to drive her to London from Essex.

My cousin Vincent is unmistakable, even after all these years, albeit obviously older and looking very drawn. There is that lean look I remember from his wedding forty years ago, with

a long face, a chin more pointed than round. Elaine had that look too, as his bridesmaid, which incidentally I had wanted to be, but was not asked. Her face is fuller now, and she looks care worn. I know she has been widowed twice since those bridesmaid days. I notice her hair is slightly messy, slightly bundled, in an attractive sort of way. Mother always had curly, untamed, hair and my daughters and I never choose what I would call neat hair. My second
daughter was an actuary before she became a mother, and in those days she said that, however smart she needed to be in her job, she always had to have slightly messy hair.

My mother had two brothers, Ernest, who was ten years older than her, and Albert, who was younger. Sitting around her bed is Ernest's oldest son Vincent, and his youngest child Elaine, who quickly tells me that the second boy, Neil, was unable to come due to his own ill health. These cousins are a lot older than any of my mother's children, and well into their retirement years.

Mother and her two brothers grew up in the East End of London. They lived behind a newsagent's shop which was owned and run by my grandmother. Little has ever been said about her husband, my mother's father. He worked in the City, was apparently sensitive, had lovely fair skin, and died in his fifties. One of the causes on the Death Certificate, according to my mother, was 'nervous debility.' Mother also told my sister, 'he had a bit of a paddy on him,' but to me he always came across as a shadowy figure, perhaps because so little is told of him. But, when I think about it, I don't know a lot about my relatives, probably because the only ones Mother talked about were her mother and her aunts.

The story I have been told is that, after Ernest was born, my grandmother did not find her husband's income from the City job enough, and so she decided to get a shop, for that had been the way of life for her and her sisters after their father died. My mother appeared when Ernest was ten years old, and was not part of my grandmother's life plan. Then Albert arrived only eighteen months later, which must have made work in the shop difficult. However, Grandmother was not going to give up, and so the children lived at the back of the shop, cared for by a series of paid 'helps.'

Ernest left and married young and my mother believed that he was put out by the arrival of two siblings after being an only child for ten years. She also thought that his early departure was caused by the shop being next door to a Fish and Chip shop, which Ernest claimed made his clothes smell permanently of fish. Whatever the reason, he married at twenty, to a woman who was more than ten years his senior. Now, here, around Mother's bed, are two of his children. It says something of the nature of my mother's recent collapse that some of the Essex part of the family have found themselves moved to travel to London for the first time in fifty years. We did all meet very recently, at the funerals of both Ernest and Albert in Essex, but before that we had not seen each other for forty years.

Mother is sitting on top of the bedcovers when we arrive, so we can all see her feet. Of course, I have always known they were bad, but have not seen them out of shoes, or at least tights, for a long while. Enormous bunions push the big toes across the rest of the toes at right angles; and I find myself thinking, who wouldn't be difficult and bad tempered with painful feet like that?

I stroke her feet and suggest, as I have many times before, that she must have had very ill fitting shoes as a child. Then we get one of the few stories re-wound of how she always had the best of everything, including being sent to a private school, and how her mother dressed her in a brown velvet dress and tied a brown velvet bow in her hair.

'She loved my hair, and was always brushing it,' she tells us all now, as if not told before, touching her hair, moving her head from side to side, as she goes on about her mother always buying the best, sending carers to buy her shoes while she stayed working n the shop. My older cousin is shaking his head at me across the bed. 'No,' his head is still going from side to side, as he whispers, almost only mouths, the words to me. 'They were neglected'.

Maybe his father was more honest with himself and his children, than my mother has been. Many children make golden a childhood that was bad, but that smell of fish must have knocked the gilt off for him.

Albert's way of coping had been different yet again. He

worked with his mother all her life, and carried on the shop after her death, though the family business had by then moved from London to Essex. His story was that grandmother was a 'muddler,' not good at business, and so not keeping the books straight. She allowed customers 'tick' and borrowing, and listened to their hard-luck stories. If someone came in for a quarter of chocolates she would open a half pound box and weigh out a quarter, in spite of the fact that she had done the same with a different box last week and
could have used up that one. Albert had got everything in order. Ernest faced reality and left. Mother was in denial, and damaged. Albert's way was to be the saviour.

Maybe my mother's damage went much deeper and she hid the anger even from herself, which could explain her lifelong enshrinement of her mum. I was later to discover that she also felt guilty about something that had happened to her mother, and I suppose if you feel guilty, how can you then complain of neglect?

When my grandmother was pregnant with Albert, she fell and broke her arm. She had left her baby girl, my mother, in a bath full of water, and was running back to her when she fell. Had she popped briefly into the shop? One can only wonder. According to my mother, the arm was never properly set, and this has been used by grandmother's daughter all her life as an excuse for everything, including the neglect. 'Mum had to work in the shop because she could not get out, because she had broken her arm.'

These cousins, around the hospital bed, I have hardly
seen, and never really talked to, and now we wait `til middle age to begin sharing family history. The bit about neglect is honest, but how deep are we prepared to go? How much time do we have? The subject is quickly changed.

'Oo, what do you do?` Elaine smiles across Mother's bed at my daughter.

'I'm a teacher.'

'Oo, that's nice. What do you teach?`

'Maths.'

'Ooo, nice. Isn't that nice?'

I have not come from a family of real intimacy where there has been real talk about real things. Certainly, there was nobody I could have turned to in my developing years. I guess such was rare in my mother's day as well as mine. Of course, I know people now who are more likely to discuss where they are going for their holidays or what they are planning to do to the house, but I also have friends who will explore with me their more complicated inner workings.

I mean spiritual workings, not the physical workings of the 'down below'- the euphemism used by my mother's generation and which covered periods, childbearing, water works, bowels and sex. Hushed references to those private secrets seem to have been the closest women those days got to anything personal, amidst the complaints about weather, buses, the rising cost of food and poor wages.

Of course, lack of money, and of cars, must have had something to do with why we cousins hardly met all our lives, but Vincent and Neil were successful college lecturers for many years, since before I grew up. Possibly the lack of extended family support lends weight to Vincent's claim of 'neglect'.

Was there any family love present in the maligning my mother received because of her 'gallivanting and frittering? Who was there for the children behind the shop? Did the paid helps pocket grandmother's money and buy cheap shoes? And I wonder what other forms of neglect, or worse, were inflicted on my mother.

*

The close death-bed experience which brought long lost relatives rushing to her bedside, has weakened Mother and put her at risk. After an attempt to let her live at home after that hospital stay – an attempt which did not work – it has been decided that she must go into Residential Care. The Social Services have long seen her increasing inability to cope with the flat. They have seen the mess in which she has lived as all part of encroaching 'dementia'. I know differently. It is yet another part of the protest. It is the rush to get out, almost as soon as she wakes each day, the running out from who knows what. To wash the dishes first or even to wash herself would have kept her in the flat longer than she could bear. Once maybe she did more of all that, but age, I grant them that, has slowed her down. Why should anyone wash dishes when there is no joy to balance it? Would Cinderella still be singing, eighty years on? And I, who have no work, why should I do some dismal job to support a life I do not even like?

Well, that is how I felt when the last divorce was finally over. It is better now, but I am still too hurt to do the one job I know I could get, in the current climate, at my age: that of Carer. And after giving up my youth in education, for something better.

And it is I who now have to clear her flat. I go there first to sort clothes for the Home, and of course they are all dirty. An egg stain on the front of this woolly, gravy spilled down that skirt. My task is made even more unpleasant by the whiff of urine which has been around my mother for years.

She did use a Council laundry service so I can face the drawer of underwear, not that she would have used the service often, or for everything. I remember always the attitude of 'it will do for another day'. When she washed things herself, including when she washed for us, she would talk of 'just rinsing' something out which when translated meant actually hardly getting it clean at all, just swirling it around in the water. From the age of eleven, I did my own washing and that of my youngest brother.

I manage to find two clean tops and one skirt, as well as enough undergarments and nightwear. A few items I can just about face washing myself, but the really dirty ones will have it be ditched and replaced.

'She shows signs of abuse,' my eldest daughter said, years ago, when she was reading for her degree in Psychology. 'It is the muckiness for a start. That is often a sign of the abused child.'

I asked my mother once, and every now and then I have tried to talk to her, about herself and her behavior. I have really tried, but it is impossible.

'She won't even know what you're talking about,' said my son when I complained of the silence. He and I both read Philosophy, as well as English, for our degrees. And of course literature is about Psychology. She has driven me mad most of my life, always accusing, criticizing, bullying, and riding rough-shod over me. Now and again I have tried to ... counsel her I suppose you could call it.

I have always been gentle, explain how hurt I have been, how damaged my self-esteem. I have assured her that I will understand if there is some problem, and that I do want to help. Then, once, I asked her if she were sexually abused as a child.

'No, nobody hurt me,' she replied.

Methinks the lady doth protest?

I have wondered about shadowy Dad too, of whom she speaks so little. I have thought of what might have gone on behind the shop, with her mum busy in there. There were always men around and about at grandmother's place, in the shop or behind it, I mean. Were they occasional shop workers, neighbours, old uncles?

Once when I was a child, I had impetigo: I had the spots all over my body, and cream had to be applied to each one. It was when I was about four, I think, or five. My mother took me to the shop and presumably told what task was before her. All my clothes were taken off and I had to stand on a kitchen chair. The memory is vague, but a man was there and he put a special cream on each spot, one by one. I felt uncomfortable and humiliated. Surely this was emotional abuse, to strip naked a child in front of anyone other than its mother, or someone in the medical profession? It was utter thoughtlessness, and whoever that man was, it felt wrong. I knew it was not right.

The outward motive was almost certainly that of wanting to help, because Mother came across as being so inadequate. Our scruffy, dirty state was testament enough of that. I have to allow that the muckiness could have had causes other than her having been abused – laziness maybe? Perhaps complete dispiritedness? All my life her slippers were trodden down at the back. For whatever reason, our mother never cared about her appearance, or that of her children. As we grew older, we two girls particularly asked for nice clothes like other girls of our age.

'You should not be interested in what you look like,' was all we got from Mother. 'I'd rather have a nice outing any day.' Secretly,

I thought, how can you enjoy a nice outing, let alone a nice holiday, if you have only rags to wear?

It was worse at school, and how we envied the girls who had neat pleated skirts, and home knitted twin-sets. They always looked so pretty, so clean, and so well cared for even envied the children who had their gloves attached to ribbon or elastic which went through their coat sleeves, so that they would never lose them and get cold hands. Their mothers cared. My hands were often blue with cold, and sometimes my fingers turned white. I now know that for life I have suffered from Raynaud's Disease, which means that in cold weather the blood runs to the vital organs and there is not enough for all the extremities.

We often had coats with hems hanging down and no buttons, and skirts which hung below the coats. I remember socks which had lost their elasticity so that they rode down into the shoes, until your foot was half uncovered and rubbing on the shoe, resulting in blisters. Once, when my feet had stopped growing, I wore the same pair of shoes everyday for eighteen months and they cut my feet until they bled. At the age of five I remember having no hanky and having to blow my thick snot onto my vest.

Yes, I was physically uncomfortable, and jealous of all those cared for children, but also I felt embarrassed and ashamed. Yet what I envied most was not the comfort and the prettiness of other girls, but that someone loved and cared enough about them to make them look pretty. I envied the ribbons and bows, which so often matched the colors of the clothes they wore.

When, during a war time air raid, we went to the Underground Station for refuge, there was sometimes entertainment. One of those entertainments was ballroom dancing, performed by a young boy and girl. The girl wore a long dress, and had a lovely bow in her long curls. A different dress and bow each time we saw them. Oh, how I wished I were that girl.

Our Dad used to comb out our tangles and then scrag our hair back into plaits, the hair on top being pulled tight and flat around the parting which made our round faces look fat. Oh, how I wanted pretty hair and fancy bows. But since my sister once had to be taken to a hairdresser to have her tangles cut out, and we both on separate occasions had our hair combed by teachers in front of a whole class of children, perhaps I can't blame my dad too much for that. Unlike little Nellie, our mum, my sister and I did not have a hair-brushing and bow-tying mother

When I was about ten, and my mother about forty, she started to wear what I called 'the dress.' This was a floral affair, dress or overall, which she wore next to her skin. She wore it day in, day out, under her nightdress at night and under her ordinary clothes in the day, so that it never came off. We didn't have baths very often and the presence of the dress said to me that she was never naked, except for that rare occasional bath.

No longer able to stand the stench of urine, I bundle the minimum of clothes into bags and close the door on Mother's flat. I had not liked to drink there, all the time I was in the smell, so as soon as I arrive at my home, I drink a half pint mug of water. My grandmother died of heart and kidney dropsy, which I know is to do with water retention. Water retention runs in the family, and I have learned that, magically, drinking pure water flushes fluid through the system and away, so I drink pints all day every day, as part of my desperate bid to escape my inheritance.

I go through my lonely evening routines of cooking,
exercising, and meditation. Then I read ten pages each of three books: Self Help, books for my Literature Class, and a detective novel. I make notes of words from my books that I will put into my 'quotes' book. Everything I do, unless I have to be somewhere else, I do in my bedroom. Of course I have to go out into the house to wash, to cook, and to clean. I go to the study to use the computer or sort through files or prepare for my writing class, or make a greetings card.

I obviously spend evenings in my bedroom, but beside that, anything I can possibly do in or on my bed, I do: reading, writing a letter by hand, writing a story, answering the telephone doing a crossword, listening to the radio, or meditating.

That night, after sorting my mother's things, my cardigan girl came to me. In a vision or a dream. I call her 'My Cardigan Girl' because she has haunted me ever since I read of her in one of Margaret Drabble's first novels.

She is a young married woman, and is described as walking down the road wearing a cardigan. She is hunched up and drags the cardigan round her bosom. Clutching it to her, she bends her head and brings her shoulders forward, making her chest seem almost concave. What is she doing? Hiding her breasts? Is she frightened that her breasts will bring her more sex, which so far has brought her a baby and unhappiness?

'Why have you come to me 'Cardigan Girl?' I ask her, and the questions come thick and fast. 'Is it to show me what 'the dress' was to my mother? Is it a sexual escape? To hide your femininity, so that no man will bother you? Are you telling me that is what my mother has been doing? Is that the meaning behind all the smelly clothes in my mother's flat?'

Chapter 3

'I want my suitcases,' Mother demands. It's my first visit to Fawsett House, and I am eager to see if Mother has settled in.

'She keeps asking for her suitcases,' the Carer tells me. 'She wants to go home.'

'They've taken my suitcases and hidden them,' she speaks fiercely. 'You've got to go and find them.'

I try to calm her down with `later` lies.

'Look, I've brought you some nice clean clothes, Mum.'

'I'm going to sue them,' she snaps back at me.

Poor Mum. Does she have any suitcases? She`s hardly been on holiday for thirty years.

'You didn't have any cases, Mum. You came here in a hurry, remember?'

'Who got me in here? That's what I want to know. I'll sue them.'

'You haven't been well, Mum.' I try to touch her, show some compassion, but she pushes me away.

'What are they talking about? I've only been a bit under the weather, that's all.`

I recall one hospital visit after the collapse that put her in here. When I arrived one day, I found a doctor trying to insert a drip into her arm. 'Isn't it a game?` she grinned at me. And, when he had gone, 'I don't know what they're messing about at.'

'You've got to get me a solicitor,' she says now, and the Carer says she'll go and get us both a nice cup of tea.

'Isn't it nice, your daughter has come to visit you,' the Carer smiles at Mum, as she leaves to make the tea.

'Nice? Nice?' My mother glares at me. 'Not if you're not going to make them give me my suitcases.'

The residents, in chairs round the room, lean and loll, either asleep or oblivious to us. They are all women and another visitor comes in who is a daughter too.

While my mother yaps on and on about her suitcases and suing somebody, my mind begins to stray and I find myself wishing that a son would come to visit a parent, a man for me, and that an old man would become a resident, an old man for Mother. Is that why you sleep, my sleeping beauties? I ask the residents in my head.

'Who got me in here? It was you, wasn't it?' She points an accusing finger at me. 'You got me in here. Why can't I come back with you?' Always the same whine, I remember the whine. The tea comes and is placed on the table between us, together with a plate of biscuits.

Mother has already got hold of one, dunked it and dropped half of that down her jumper, when a son does come in. He nods across to me, and comes over to speak. Am I new here – or rather is my mother, ha ha? He needs to talk, and explains how his mother deteriorated very suddenly. He shows me a picture of a totally different woman taken just two years ago. He stands quite close, showing me the photograph. He is a good looking man. Mother leans forward to sort through the biscuit selection. She does it aggressively and makes the table shake. My cup joggles so I pick it up. Mother is annoyed and ratty, as she is not getting the attention she has always demanded of me.

'You might show me the photograph first,' she snaps. The man smiles at me, and leans towards her, but she turns sharply and tries to grab the photo, knocking my cup sideways.

My cup spilleth over. And I have hot tea from lower stomach to upper leg.

*

Weeks later it is still going on. 'Haven't you brought my suitcases?' Demands for suitcases, threats about suing somebody, and attacks on me for getting her into this Home.

Her Social Worker took her back to her flat one day, and asked her if she really wanted to go back. Faced with the reality, Mother said, 'no'. It is a cheerless place, and the sight of it must have brought back memories of the loneliness which drove her out, dying, to her beloved riverside.

To enable the authorities to keep someone in Residential Care, they have to get permission from the clients themselves, unless of course the person is sectioned. That is not only a difficult thing to do, but it is never a permanent order, and can be revoked at anytime. So, I find myself back in the urine stench to do more clearing out. I am not going to clear the flat completely. Why should it always be me? I will find a house clearance company, or the Council. It is a Council owned property, after all, and they are in a hurry for vacant possession.

Fawsett House has asked that I bring things she treasures and anything that might help to make her feel more at home, like a favourite armchair. I smile to myself. I doubt that she values anything in her home. She has never been a home lover. I bash through the rooms, filling bags with out-and-out rubbish.

There are bits of food all over the kitchen, in cupboards, in the fridge, and covering all the surfaces. There are half finished tins, opened packets, food that has gone off or is well out of date. A mug is crammed full of used tea-bags. Once, I threw out all the everlasting tea bags and when I returned the next day the mug was full again. There was no way there had been time for her to have drunk that much tea. Her statement was clear, 'I am in control, and nobody makes the decision about when to throw the tea-bags out but me.'

Everywhere I see these instances of those who have control over so little, clutching tightly on to whatever small areas they can find. I reflect, as I have done many times before, that none of us can have control over everything, and even that sometimes it does not matter. We can let control go when there is something else more important. It surely matters only that we stand firm about important issues? Very insecure people will exert a rigid control over anything and everything, even at their own expense, like filling their home with these squashed, 'dead-mice,' tea-bags.

No, my mother has never valued any home she has had, and always spent the minimum time looking after it. As with nice clothes, the answer was always the same, 'I'd rather have a nice outing.' She has never picked up a paint brush or papered a wall, and if anyone else did it for her she would complain about the mess and the upheaval.

A few times my dad did do a bit of decorating, and used what people in the post war days did – a paint called 'distemper'– which was always yellow in colour and cheap. How he had the time or the money for even that, I do not know. Some years later, Mother's youngest brother, Albert, came and helped Dad put up some much needed kitchen cupboards, for kitchens in those days were often equipped with little more than a stove, a sink and a small table for working on. Mother could not stand the noise, the mess, the activity – the disruption she called it – and got out of the place as much as possible. 'Men like banging and making a mess,' she has always said about all men embarking on any kind of

D.I.Y. Despite this, she was forever whining to me about other people's 'nice houses.' Did she think it was just there, the nice house, bought like that because you had money and that money brought the magic of nothing ever needing replacing or refurbishing? As soon as I was old enough, I cleared up myself if I wanted friends to tea. I bought material with the money from my holiday job, and made curtains and cushion covers.

I look around her flat now, and see there is a rut from the bed to bathroom where the morning trail of unchecked urine has gnawed at the carpet. Once, the Council came to do something about the smell, but she shoo-ed the man away and slammed the door. The incontinence pads were delivered by a Social Service team, who also collected the used ones, but sometimes she denied that she had any, sent them away empty handed, and days later they were found by the Home Help, hidden at the back of her wardrobe.

Oh sad, sad souls who can no longer have secrets. I am told that, already, in the Home she hides her dirty underwear.

I decide I am not staying in this smell any longer. I'll take the footstool to the Home, and the corner unit. This has lots of little shelves for ornaments and photographs. A woman who used to live in the flats gave it to her, and she did like that neighbour.

Photographs, they are one of the things she may like. I look around desperately. No, I am definitely going to leave all the furniture. One of the family members may like the gate- leg table, and even Dad's old record player. I'll tell them they've got three days to come and collect. The smaller things I can take home to sort. I have already been through the jewellery, cosmetics and toiletries and taken these to her. Magically, she seems to have had the powder compact with her from the start. She would not be without that, with its pressed powder foundation and little mirror. She loves her compact.

So, the next major job is the paperwork. I hold my breath for as long as it takes to locate letters, photographs, papers and cards, bundle them into a bag and get out to my car quickly. There are a few framed photos of her brothers and her mother that she will like to have round her, and some of us. There is not one of my dad.

*

Mother's childhood home was the East End of London, and the most usual place of recreation from there for days out and longer holidays was Southend. Here, Mother told me, she met our Dad. It was at the permanent funfair, which was called the Kersel. She was twenty-seven and he twenty-four. My father liked women, or maybe it would be truer to say that he liked sex. Future events revealed him as pretty randy, and it could be said irresponsibly so, like taking me to see a show with one of his other women.

My mother, undoubtedly, would have been very attractive to him. We have heard all our lives about the glorious hair, which her mother loved to brush. It was auburn, or Titian as she called it, and very thick and curly. I have been told that it caused people to turn their heads to look when she walked down the street. She also had big breasts. It seemed she put a lot of care into her appearance in those days. She always had the Mason Pearson hairbrush, which bore testament to her always having the best. She wore Kaiser Bondar brassieres, and an aunt taught her to finish washing her face by splashing it with cold water. She insists on doing that to this day, even in Fawsett House.

I do not know exactly how it came about, but she conceived my eldest brother very soon after meeting my dad. She told me when I was a teenager that she did not know how babies came about until she was having one herself.

As I grew up, I soon noticed that my school friends had pictures of their parents' weddings in their houses. 'Why haven't we got a wedding photograph, of you and Dad?' asked my mother when I was about eight years old.

'Oh, it was in the war,' she replied. 'Lots of people didn't bother. We didn't take photographs in those days.' I was confused because we had pictures of my eldest brother as a baby, and he was born in the war.

'How long were you married, before you had Victor?'
asked a bit later. It was an innocent question, probably romantic because by then I had watched films where people got married, then sometime later had a child.

'Oh, two years,' Mother replied quickly. I asked her what she had worn for her wedding and she told me that it was a silver grey suit, which was what most brides wore. The 'two years' and 'silver grey suit' were stereotypical answers – as if she were telling someone else's story.

When I was eleven I needed my Birth Certificate as part of my entrance for an examination to obtain a place at a grammar school. My mother told me where to look for it, in the big box where it was kept with other important papers. As I searched through the papers, my eyes were not taking much in. I was intent on seeing the words Birth Certificate and then seeing if I had the one with my name on it. However, the words Marriage Certificate did catch my eye. I had never seen an official document before, so naturally I was curious. I read through it and discovered the first shock when I read, after my father's name, the words, 'formally married to Gwendoline, from whom he obtained a divorce.' Then I saw the date of the wedding. My parents had married two weeks before my eldest brother was born. This has never been discussed openly in the family. I did not tell anybody at the time, and it was only decades later that my younger brother told me he had the same experience and shock. He too needed to search for his Birth Certificate when a child, and made the same discovery as I did. We children never asked our parents about this. At some stage, I learned that Dad had a daughter with Gwendoline, Margaret, but I know nothing of him keeping in touch with her or supporting her. I suppose this lack of talking in my immediate family stemmed from the lack of real communication in the wider one.

Bit by bit, I have pieced together the story from other relatives. My mother discovered that she was pregnant, was sent to an Unmarried Mothers' Home, and my father forced by her family to marry her. But it took him until the eleventh hour to get his divorce finalised.

So there are no photographs of my father in any of the frames in my mother's flat and I wonder why. I have been flicking through one of the old photograph albums, seeing my parents with us, so many of which were taken on the beach at Southend. Our early family life was spent in the East End too, and later we moved to a village only a few miles from the East Enders' seaside resort.

The smell of urine hits my nostrils again, and this time it sickens me. It seems it is on everything I handle. I cannot do any more sorting out of photographs letters and cards, so I go out to my shed, which is falling to bits and therefore airy, and put the boxes of Mother's papers in there. Maybe some of the smell will blow away, I hope.

Standing in the shed, I hear a rat-tat on the front door. I peep round the garden gate and see my son in the drive, at my front entrance, which is at the side of the house.

'Hello duck,' he says. This is one of our 'in jokes' and is an eternal memorial to my mother, as she often calls people 'duck.'

'Just passing,' says Rafe. As a Gilbert and Sullivan fan, I gave him the name of a character in one of their works. I think my three girls could be relieved that they are not Mabel, Elsie and Ida!

'Come to see what jobs you've got for me. I might be able to do some on Saturday,' he says. I make him tea, and offer him what all the children come to me for, my homemade flapjack. I still have some of Mother's stuff on the table, 'Who's that?' he asks curiously, and begins questioning me on one of the open photograph albums. I fill him in on a bit of family history but have to own up that I do not know who half the people are.

'Doesn't she look young?' I point to my mother's cousin who I know to be already older, than I am now, in that snapshot. She looks half her age. He studies the photograph. 'Yes, but it is a war-time face, isn't it?' He says, and now I realise how often I have noticed that every age, each era, has its own `face.' I first noticed this in a friend of my age who looked like a forties film star, and thought she must somehow have been born out of time. What I worked out then was that some families must have very big gaps between all generations, which was why a girl of thirty looked like a forties movie star in 1970. My mother's cousin would have a war time face, but my son pointing it out reminds me that each age does have a face, albeit some, like my friend, don't fit into that.

I like the way my son always gives his full attention to anything I show or tell him, and does not dismiss it with any glib comment. He often notices things that I don't. We go on to discuss what is the most pressing of my jobs. Nearly every time Rafe turns up it's the same, 'I've come to do jobs.'

The shed is falling down and that is only half the story. I am not long out of a short, second marriage to a 'con' man, and lost half my assets. I lost my work too, what with the nature of the divorce, then the recession. Only with the help of my children do I keep myself teetering along regarding the house and garden 'jobs.' The times I feel nearest to suicide is when I come home and see all that needs to be done in the house and garden, work which I have neither the energy nor the money to address. Then there is the cleaning. I have increasingly less heart for that.

I think if anyone knew that I live in my bedroom – on my bed – they would call it going back to the womb. What I remember is that I gradually retreated there, choosing that over any alternative, because the room is the brightest and warmest in the house, and the bed the most comfortable place

After we have made a list of Saturday's jobs my son goes, and I put aside the photographs I will take to Mother tomorrow.

*

'Have you brought the suitcases?' Mother greets me as I arrive. My heart sinks lower and it seems that it is going to be another difficult visit. The words come quickly; she does not want to be here. She demands suitcases and solicitors, and keeps on that she is going to sue somebody.

I try to distract her by showing her the photographs, but she pushes them away. Tea is brought in, but as there is no man near me, I doubt I'll get burnt this time. My poor beauties lean and loll. They are asleep, all but one. She walks up and down, up and down, and in and out. She comes into the room where we sit, out again, then she comes back in, and this time goes out into the garden. It is still summer, yet she wears a winter coat. The walking legs are mottled with sores, above thick striped socks and battered trainers. The others loll as she walks, and I pick up the photographs again, beginning to direct my mother's attention to them, one by one.

'Look, here's your mum,' I say. 'And here is the outside of the shop.' She doesn't say anything, so I continue. 'What was it like? What was it like, your childhood?'

'I just wished I had an ordinary mum,' she says.

'What do you mean?'

'I used to wish that I had a cosy mum, one who did not have to be in the shop.'

'Did you feel a bit neglected then?' I hazard. The reaction is fierce. Her mother was good to her. She was always brushing her hair, tying on the velvet bow, and giving her the best of everything. She touches her hair, turning her head from side to side. 'She sent me to a private school you know, only me. I sometimes wonder if the boys resented it.' But she did not like school, she goes on. She could not do the sums and was very nervous.

'I just wished I had a mum like the other children, who could meet me from school, like theirs did.'

Going through the photographs, I came upon one of my dad, in the garden of Grandmother's shop, on the arm of a nurse, presumably from the Nurses' Home that I had heard was across the road from the shop. They were smiling into each other's eyes. I quickly put that one at the back of the pile and point out a picture of her youngest brother, the one near her age, wondering what this will bring out. 'Oh, he and I always got into such scrapes.' She is lighter now, laughing. 'Always up to mischief, that was us. Sitting on the upstairs window ledges and frightening our mother to death. All I can ever remember of him is being tucked under someone's arm and taken to the Nurses' Home over the road, next door to the pub. He seemed to be always cutting his head or something.'

My grandmother's name was Mildred, but she was always called Jack. Was she one of the first of the modern women, I wonder? Years ago, in the days when the chant that 'you're a cabbage if you stay at home' sent so many of us out to do cabbagy jobs, I used to wonder if my mother were some kind of warning of what could happen to the child of the mother who worked.

I pick up another photograph of the two brothers together, and she begins to wail that they are both now 'gone'. At least she knows that, and remembers it, if only for this moment. When I met her at the hospital, my cousin Elaine said to me, 'I think the boys put her down a little bit.' From a family which has never been nurturing in my experience, and has mostly maligned my mother – with the 'gallivanting and frittering' – this was quite something. I think that the two brothers must have put her down rather a lot. Maybe that is why she is as she is. All my life she has beaten herself with sticks because 'I can't knit,' or 'I have never made a cake,' and has been completely untouched by my saying that lots of women can't and don't.

I think of her brothers and how it must have been for two young males of that generation to find themselves in a household where the most dominant member was a female - their mother. They could not punish her. Apart from how would they, men – and most of us perhaps – tend to enshrine mothers, but all that hate had to go somewhere. Any resentment left over from their mothering, men usually take out on their wives, girl friends or women colleagues. But these two had a handy smaller female in their childhood home, who maybe was already half damaged by then, and so a ready victim.

'... I used to get fed up, behind the shop.' I have not been listening, thinking of the brothers. 'Every now and then I would pack up my things, get on the tram, and turn up on Auntie Nellie's doorstep.' As with the velvet bow, I know the rest of the story already.

'What are you doing here? ` Auntie Nellie would say.

'I've come to stay,' my mother would reply.

'Well, you'd better come in then.'

It is only now that something about this story hits me, and it has never occurred to me before. I turn to Mother. 'I thought Auntie Nellie had a shop too?` What I had always heard was that Jack did not have time for my mother because she was always in the shop.

'Oh yes, but she was different. She didn't have any children.' So, could she make time because it was not constant? Or was she more motherly?

I begin to pack up the photographs, asking which ones she would like to have in her room, whether there are any of the loose ones she would like me to frame. She is tired. She is called Nellie too. She has always hated the name, and I am wondering whether, had she been called Eleanor, things would have been different, when another relative comes in. One of the other sleeping beauties does indeed wake with a kiss, a daughterly kiss.

Even my mother livens. 'I haven't seen her before,' she says, and the two nod and smile across to us. Since we are the only four people awake in the place, daughter helps her mother over to join us, on her walking frame. While the two older ladies chat, I learn that daughter is in fact daughter-inlaw. Her husband, the older lady's son, died two years ago, and it was the shock of his death which put his mother into Residential Care. Daughter-in-law appears to be younger that me, but has a moustache.

The sleepers sleep on, and the walker comes and goes. We talk for a bit before the older ladies grow tired. It is time to go. I quickly use the visitor's toilet near the entrance and run to my car. I have a car, which I run at great expense to every other area of my life. I use it sparingly, parking way outside towns in order not to have the further cost of parking fees. I learned to drive when I saw my mother being ferried about one Christmas, dependent on other people and obliged to leave when they wanted to go home. As I drive home, my car still smells of urine, and when I go out to my shed I find the smell has not cleared from there either. At least it won't reach as far as my bedroom, where I mostly stay.

I decide to leave the sorting of the rest of the papers until tomorrow. It is the day that I usually write to Imogen. After doing my yoga exercises, and squeezing my pelvic floor, I look at my face in the mirror as I rub in my night cream, and think how hard some women work to look beautiful. Do they do it to be loved by a man? I know I do, though I have not had much joy in that area. I do not have a moustache, and am not fat. I am good looking, and yet I have never been truly loved, and certainly have never been ravished, as I would like to be.

Then I understand the moustache lady. She is a young widow – alone, but perhaps it is less painful not to try, than to try and fail. Better not to look as though you are in the game, than for it to be obvious to all, and to you, that you are not winning. Better to jump off the roundabout. Better to stay in the glass case.

I go to sleep thinking of the moustache lady, but dream of the Cardigan Girl. She walks up and down, up and down.

Chapter 4

Sorting through my mother's things, I come upon a postcard, and remember Worthing. It has not been sent to her, it hasn't even been written on. She must have bought it while visiting the place, and brought it back to remind her. Sometimes she did send postcards, including to me or my children, when she had only a day trip to the seaside. She even bought seaside rock for the children. She had few enough actual holidays. In her last active years, Worthing has always been her first choice, and I have taken her there myself many times.

Why do I do all this sorting out for Mother? Why have I seen her at least once a week since I left home, whatever my family or health condition – even work – may have been? Why, in her last five years, did I take her out all day every Sunday? The answer is simple: because I thought I had to, that`s all.

'I don't see why it should be you, every week,' a friend once said to me.

'Well, it is something to do with the day,' I replied, 'and she does buy me a meal.' If I am true, what else was there for me to do, other than take her out? It has only been since that last marriage and divorce, which so shattered me, that I began taking her out every Sunday. It has come to me that her vision may have been so strong, so straight lined and single minded, that I would be providing for her to the end, that on some deeper level she created that. Created the low self image which has ended me here with no work, no partner, and living round the corner from her.

Nothing I have done has ever been enough, and she would say to everyone, 'she only takes me out once a week.' Yet it was hardly my fault – the gypsy caravan or the camper van, I mean. But I think she thinks it is. Yet, sometimes I would wonder as I looked across the restaurant table at her on our Sunday outings, at that look of abject misery, wonder if it were staged, for my benefit. I think about the caravan and the camper van and wonder why she has never been abroad. She has never had much of an income, and of course there has been the frittering, but I can't help thinking that, if it was her greatest desire, she might have done it once, just once.

Saved the sixpences in a jar, joined a holiday club, done something. The look across the table would say to me, 'look how miserable I am. You can't dare to be happy, could not surely bear to be happy, with a mother as wretched as I am.' Did she purposely not go abroad so that I would keep the ball and chain I received as a child, unable to attend to my own life, until I had provided for hers? Her saving the sixpences would have been like me going to Dating Agencies. I have never got the equivalent pay out of the holiday – the happy relationship – but at least I tried and `saved the sixpences`. Sometimes I am filled with horror when I think of the time I have given to my mother. Where were my children, what were they doing? She never wanted them around. She only wanted me.

When my third child was born, she said to me, 'Oh, don't have anymore babies,' and I knew she did not say it out of concern for my finances, my lifestyle, or even my health. It is strange this syndrome of separating mothers from their children, of wanting the mother to yourself. I call it the Rumpelstiltskin syndrome because I sense that it is more than wanting the mother's attention for you. It is enjoying the cruelty of separating the mother and child, as Rumpelstiltskin did. What other motive could there be for him choosing the price he did, other than one of cruelty?

To separate a parent from a child, is that the greatest hatred, revenge for something on someone and so on the world? I wonder if, secretly, in human hearts it is known that the greatest prize really is a child -- a golden joy..

I have known men who are Rumpelstiltskins too. They shut the door of the room where they sit with their women, and keep the children out. They take their women out at the weekend on some errand which 'will only take half an hour,' and then it takes three.

While my children were young, weekends for Mother meant visiting us, not trips out. I sat alone with Mother. The children played in other rooms. She would have criticized them if they had been there. Once, after a Mother's Day spent like this, and with time broken up by elevenses, lunch and tea, I finally walked her to her bus at the end of the day, and we even had a pub drink with crisps on the way. When I got back in doors I ate and ate and ate, even though I had been eating all day.

Eating has always been the way we have spent our Sundays during the last five years. By then I had a car and we drove to a coffee place, on to a pub lunch, then to a supermarket for shopping, and tea. I tried to make sure that one of those stops was by water or by trees, but it was the meals that provided the framework for the day.

*

What else was there to do with Mother but eat? I thought that day in Worthing. We had just arrived by coach and there is a café round the corner from the Coach Station, and opposite the sea, where we always start our day. I looked round at the plastic tables, plastic chairs, and plastic food. The placer reminded me of the old Milk Bars of my childhood.

Forever watching my diet, my weight, and my purse, I rarely have a cake. On such a day as this, I always feel I deserve one – and Mother is urging and begging me to let her buy me a cake – but all it seems I can see is plastic lemon meringue pie. Not worth getting fat for.

'I used to come here for the day,' Mother says. 'By coach, when you were all at school.' Another day trip on the coach, I think to myself. 'A couple of times I stayed a few days,' she continues. I don't recall, but maybe by then I was married, and she only had the younger two at home. Did she leave them, as she makes me leave my children? 'The only trouble was the evenings. I got lonely. Once I telephoned Dad. ` But I always made a bee-line for this place, as soon as I got here. I thought it was glamorous.` The back wall is completely covered in a poster of Italy, of a foreign place.

Glamorous!'

*

I look at the postcard again, and think of that tatty place which spoke glamour to her. Will taking this to Fawsett House cheer her up as she remembers, or will it remind her that it was the nearest she ever got to glamour – or to the camper van?

I put it on the 'not sure pile'. I have done enough for this evening.

So did my mother crave glamour? Was that the cause of her malaise? This word, in her description of the Worthing café, opens a different file of slides in my memory. First, the woman in a book about Death Row, that examines the lives of the prison inmates, and shows how so often abuse, either private or social, almost exonerates their capital crimes. The night before the execution, a prisoner is interviewed. This particular woman has been the only character who has stayed with me since I read the book twenty years ago. For at the end of the interview she says, 'I never had a dress worth more than five dollars.'

She fades away, and I doze or dream, and now, as on the television screen where I met her, I see clearly the woman in a head scarf. Like my last visitor, she is sitting in an office, but this time her interview is about her medical treatment. It has not worked and there is no more that can be done. A doctor tells her that she has only two months to live. 'So,' says the young woman wistfully. 'I will never drive to France in an open car. Never drive to France with my hair flying.'

I sleep, but wake panting with horror, and still a scream of women seems to be rattling railings at me and asking to be heard. I remember a friend who had been threatened with divorce for her wifely shortcomings, by a husband who was not without his own, particularly in the region of being the main provider. 'I screamed at him,' she told me. 'So, I don't cook and clean well enough, eh? I don't know how to control the children? Well I will soon be thirty, and I have never worn an evening dress.'

The lovely dress, that drive in a sports car. Don't we all want to be a princess? If not to lovers then to our parents, or to someone?

The slides continue to flicker on my screen as I go through my day. Washing and dressing I look at myself and feel again the emptiness that nobody has ever really looked on me with love.

*

Today I am to take my daughter's little girl to and from school, because her regular Carer is sick. Anna teaches three days a week, and leaves for school at 7.30am in the morning, getting home nearly an hour after her child needs picking up. As I walk around the building, waiting for the bell to summon the children in, I am suddenly looking into the school hall and I am a child of five again.

It is nearly Christmas and we have played this game many times. There is a chair in the middle of the hall, and instead of the gym lesson we children are expecting we are separated into groups. The chair is a Christmas tree and we are the decorations, the candles, the balls or the parcels. When the balls are signalled, they bounce up to the chair, dance around it, then stand in position. Next, it is the turn of the children who are the candles and they join their hands in a point above their heads like flames as they dance to 'decorate' the tree. The parcels jump along to the tree with arms across their chests, like tying string. I am always the parcel. Each week a different girl is chosen to be the fairy doll and when the tree is completely decorated, she dances and stands on the chair – the Christmas tree. I am never the fairy doll.

As I drive home from the school I think of my life to date. I have been married twice. Both times I wore white and walked in last when all the church 'decorations' were in their places. Both marriages ended in divorce. Did I marry just because I wanted to be the fairy doll?

Going through my day, I keep thinking of my 'parcel' days, until another school memory comes to me, another memory of not being the chosen one. In fact this time I was not chosen at all, not even to be a parcel. Again it was nearly Christmas. I was eleven by now and I felt we should be working hard for the 'scholarship' examination, to win a place at a grammar school. The top class was to produce a Christmas play, and what I remember is that I was the only child without a part. In my memory, the whole school day was spent rehearsing this play, and I sat alone in the desks while the others performed at the front of the classroom. I soon knew every word and every part of that play, and secretly hoped that somebody would be ill on the day, but no-one was. I thought I had not been chosen because I was poor and scruffy, or fat. I was not the cherished girl with the string on her gloves, the pleats in her skirt, or the hand knitted twin-set and the bows. Maybe glamour to me was the outward sign of being cherished.

My 'war-time face' relative said to me recently. 'My husband will give me anything I want.' I have never experienced that sort of love, and felt envious. Then I remembered a quote I wrote in my `Quotes` book. I found it in a novel by Katherine Mansfield and it says, 'I suppose it's the savage pride of the female who likes to think that the man to whom she had given herself must be a very great chief indeed.'

It has been a hard day for me emotionally, and taking Molly to school, visiting those memories, has taken its toll, so I take a sleeping pill. The thoughts race through my mind, I have not the outward sign of glamour, which to me would be a sign to the world that I am an adored woman, a woman cherished and ravished.

More nightmares continue to haunt me, and I see the electric chair lady. She walks round and round a wooden school chair. Her arms are folded across her chest, and she is wearing a woolly cardigan.

Chapter 5

'I want to know what they've done with my suitcase.' Mother's voice is aggressive as I approach her today. Can't I do something about finding her suitcase? I calm her down with `later` lies, and show her the picture of Worthing. This brings me fresh trouble, as she demands to know when I am going to take her there again. I weakly pacify her by agreeing to stay for lunch. I do sometimes eat with her at the Home. What else is there to do with her but eat? The greetings are always the same, and are beginning to wear me down. She wants her suitcases, they are wicked to keep her here, and she is going to sue somebody. I must get a solicitor, and I must get her out of here. She is so depressed, but I know that has been the case for...forever.

'Some people are a bit strict about table manners,' she says, dropping her gravy down her cardigan.

'Were they with you? I ask, hoping to open up a conversation about her childhood.

'No, it was this friend Dorothy. They used to want me to come over and play with her. She was an only child, and sometimes I stayed all day, had my dinner there. They wanted company for her.'

'And they were strict with her?` I question. 'What do you mean? Rapping her over the knuckles for spilling her gravy?' 'No, making her hold her knife and fork a certain way. You know, strict.' Who was this Dorothy? All the years and I`ve never heard the name before.

'She lived over the road. They had the pub, you know.'

Now the pub, I have heard of that, many times, along with the brown velvet bow and the broken arm, and the brother with the cut head. I have heard the story over and over again, of how depressing life was in the shop, and how my mother was put off marriage, and of the young wives who would come into the shop for their husband's newspaper. How heavy she felt looking out of the living room window, which was above the shop, at the pub which was opposite.

Beautiful Dreamer

'All I saw was these poor wives, in their aprons, going into the pub to drag their husbands out for their Sunday dinner.' These stories she has told me over and over again. This was one world for her. The pub, the road, the shop and the poor wives, they all went together: the poor wives coming into the shop to buy their husband's newspaper – ` come for `is paper`– as Mother always quoted.

Not that there were no other worlds, as time went by. Mother has described the family's acquisition of a radio, in her childhood, as 'opening up another world' for her. She loved the BBC accent, 'those lovely voices,' she would say. 'It made me realise there were other worlds too,' she would say. 'I loved the radio .'

She always longed for a more cultured voice, though hers was not `East End.' It is only much later I come to realise that she had a very large vocabulary. I think she had a feel for language, maybe an affinity with it, as I do. She had he own quaint words, too, like `nobby` or `dinky` for anything small, handy, well designed. And she amused us with her ` ooer`, and `ducks`.

The cinema was yet another world for her, for the family did go to the 'pictures.' What comes across to me now is that she loved seeing beautiful ladies, like Hedy Lamarr, with the beautiful cheekbones. It is interesting because, in my childhood, she would sometimes draw sketches and they were always only of ladies, side views, and showing profiles and cheekbones. Later, the films she loved best were 'Genevieve,' and 'The Yellow Rolls Royce,' films about cars, trips out, and holidays. There has always been a thirst for adventure in my mother's desire for travel. She always had a 'wanderlust' as she put it, perhaps adventure, and that links with the only book she ever mentions from her childhood, 'The Three Musketeers', for as well as the radio and films, she loved books. She tells me that she was always reading, always had her nose in a book, and that her dad used to say she would read a piece of sugar paper. She read her favourite book many times.

Adventure and glamour too, these were in the worlds in which she escaped to in her books and in her films, the lovely places, cultured voices, smart ladies, when all the time the reality was the street outside, the shop, and the poor wives. The reality was no glamour.

When I have taken her to see a film in recent years, she has fidgeted and talked all through it. She always complained that these films were not like the old ones, the one exception being 'Mrs Doubtfire' when she laughed and laughed.

When our family got a television set in 1955, she loved it and watched it, but rarely when our father was watching. He would sit in the living room above the shop, where the television was, and she would sit in the 'kitchen' behind the shop and do her pools or write letters. She wrote to anyone she could think of about her terrible life, to see if they would help her. She even wrote to the Queen. Dad went to bed early because of getting up for work at four, and then she watched alone.

Now, in Fawsett House, she will not watch television, because it would mean sitting with the other residents. Mother always liked best to watch by herself. Anyone who did sit with her when she was intent on a television programme noticed that she would make faces as she watched. It seemed as if she were mimicking the expressions and emotions of the screen characters. Was that the closest she got to expressing her own real feelings?

Her reading has dwindled over the last twenty years, and now I cannot get her to read at all. I hunt out large print books for her, but it makes no difference. Almost anything I offer her to have or to do, she pushes away. They have singsongs and visiting entertainers in the Home, but she will not join in.

So now we have this Dorothy. Somehow the meal I am having with Mother in the Home has jogged her memory about dinners with Dorothy, and how the girl's parents were strict with her about table manners. But then she goes back to the poor wives.

'They all had the white weddings,' she says. 'The white dress, the flowers, the veils. They loved their veils. Then in no time at all you saw them in their aprons, with their stomachs sticking out.' All my life, whenever I have been with her and we pass a wedding, or if I have talked about arranging one of my daughters' weddings, whenever there is any talk of wedding dresses or veils, it is the same retort from Mother, 'I always think of what comes after the wedding.' And I say what I have always said in reply to this. 'But you know there are other marriages, good ones, happy. Not just those of the poor wives. What about your mum and dad?'

She has never replied to this question, but many times I have heard her talk of her mother's sister Amy. 'Oh Amy was so happy, her Bert was a lovely man. Then she woke and found him dead one day. He was only thirty-nine. She said her heart was broken forever and she never got over it.'

'What about Aunty Amy?' I remind her now, and 'What about Auntie Nellie?' There is total silence. We finish our dinner and the pudding is brought by a Carer. I try again. 'Tell me about your aunties. What about your childhood?'

'I just wished I could have had a cosy mum, one who did not have to go in the shop.' 'What did you do? Who did you play with? What about the people your mum got to help? Didn't you say you had a cleaner? Mrs Roper?'

'Oh, she didn't have time for us. She always brought her children with her.'

'Did Mrs Roper have children then? Did she drag them with her, charring?

'Oh, she had umpteen children. One a year, I would think.'

'And they couldn't play with you?'

'No, they just seemed like loads of babies to me, always one more baby'.

'What did she do with them while she cleaned? Were they in a pram or something?'

'She used to tie them up.'

'Tie them up?

'To a big chair. So they wouldn't get in the way of her cleaning.'

'What did she tie them up with?' a Carer has been ear- wigging near by

'What did Mrs. Roper tie her babies up with, while she cleaned?

`A rope?`

I am momentarily stunned that my mother calls the insistence on table manners being strict, but does not blink at children being tied up. Mother is wittering on.

`.. Mr. Roper used o come and collect her sometimes. A nice, smart, dapper gentleman.`

Of course he was. I bet he was. But I want to hear about this new one, Dorothy.

'And did you go to play with Dorothy a lot?'

'They always seemed to want me to. She was an only child, you see.' So Mrs Pub Lady could not have been one of the poor wives, I observe.

'What did you play? With Dorothy, I mean. In their flat above the pub?'

'Oh we used to dress up in her mother's clothes.' Acting the fine lady of the film world, instead of the dreaded future of the poor wife and the apron I think, but Mother has remembered something else.

'There used to be a dentist……' She is now spilling custard down her front. 'He used to go in there.'

'Used to go in the pub?'

'No upstairs. To see them, you know.'

'What, he did their teeth at home?'

'No.' Mother is having difficulty with the pastry of the apple pie because we are still waiting for her new set of bottom teeth. 'There used to be talk.' She lowers her voice to the tone used by that generation for the 'down below' talk, and looks around to see that no one is listening. '…About the dentist always being in there. Some said that Dorothy was not her Father's.'

So, Mrs. Pub Lady was definitely not a poor wife then

Mrs. Pub lady had clothes worth dressing up in.

Maybe Mrs. Pub Lady even knew glamour!

Chapter 6

All these meals with Mother at the Home make me think of my mother and her relationship with food. As with the submission and rebellion, the scruffiness opposed to the cold water face splashing and the powder compact, there is this ambivalence with her and food too. On the one hand, food seems almost to be an obsession with her. Nearly always, when she meets any of her children, the question is the same. 'Have you had your food?' Not have you had your dinner, or have you had your tea? She says this every time to my youngest brother, who has never married and who she thinks should not be catering for himself.

This question would obviously only be asked if the meeting with her children were not centred round a meal, for example, when we took her out to any evening concert and she wanted to know if we had had time for our dinner. Meals in our homes, or in a restaurant, she loved, but she always wanted more than was provided. She would ask for a cup of tea when everyone was drinking wine, or for a plate of bread and butter to go with her dinner.

Most of my adult life, and particularly when I had young children, Mother always visited with offerings of food, special- offer grocery items, or broken biscuits. Once, when the children were at school, she gave me a cake, which she said was for my eldest daughter only. 'See that she gets it, and make sure she knows that it is from me.' I suppose by giving it to Anna and denying me and my other children, she was doing what she did to herself. She loved herself by taking herself out to have a cake in a café, but at other times denied herself food. During our childhood she hardly seemed to eat at all, unless in a tea shop.

*

I remember childhood tea-times with Mother. I can see her now, running in and out to where we all sat round the table after school. She does not sit with us, but runs in with food, runs out with dirty dishes, then washes up, eating the bits off our plates. We sit in what is called the kitchen, though it's more like a living room. The cooker and sink are in another room, which is called a scullery. It is the only private room downstairs behind the shop, and the living room is upstairs. By the time I was a teenager we had moved to Greater London, near Kingston upon Thames, and our accommodation was attached to the shop my father managed. It is the same as the kitchen and scullery in our last home, which was a private house and had sitting and dining rooms in the front. It was as if the 'kitchen' had moved with us. Here, as there, a fireplace stands in the kitchen, with washing always in front of it to dry. The same mantelpiece seems to have moved with us too. It is crowded with a clock, a pot of spills for Dad's pipe, postcards, a letter rack full of out of date letters and bills, a comb, a hairbrush full of hair, and possibly a vase, also full of rubbish. Anything seems to be put on the mantelpiece, like nappy pins, or a bottle of medicine.

The table is covered as always by a tablecloth, which is dirty. And, also as always, Mother is running in and out of the scullery to the kitchen. She has her hat on, as she has only just arrived back from gallivanting. She throws her shopping onto the table, still in paper bags – like a few tomatoes, or a bun round. Keeping her hat on seems to me to be saying that she wishes she were still out, or is inwardly ready to fly off again. And so she flies from scullery to kitchen, from kitchen to scullery with the big knife in her hand. It is the meat knife, but it is used for cutting bread, and she runs in to cut the bread, then back out to warm up tinned spaghetti or pasties, back in then back out to eat the leftovers. The knife is stained and she runs with it pointing outwards, like a sword.

Years later a school friend who visited often, commented that our teas were not poor. She noticed that there was always cheese and often freshly bought tomatoes. I suppose more thrifty mothers would have made cakes, and given their children just bread and jam after school. I always thought of us as poor, and I do not remember dinners very much other than school ones or those we had in cafés. Our clothes were poor and our home shabby.

Then one day, as a young teenager, I got a shock, an inward eye opener, if you like. When I was at grammar school, I went one weekend to stay with my school friend, Sandra. We stayed in her house or wandered round the shops, but we did not have a lot to do, so I suggested we went to the pictures. We called on my mother first and she gave me half-a-crown, which was more than I needed, and would buy an ice cream as well.

Sandra's mother had had to go that Saturday to the kitchen where she normally worked just in the week, so we had to go there to get some money from her. I was fascinated at the woman's reaction to her daughter's request. She looked worried at first, asked me the exact cost of a ticket to see a film, then counted that amount in pennies into the girl's hand. It made me think about the different ways people spend money, and I began to wonder just how much it would cost to buy a new school blouse, or a pair of knickers.

Now, I know that my mother was not good with money, did not budget or juggle money around so that she could afford things, and she always had the money for the pictures, but never put the sixpences in a jar for holidays. My friend's mother obviously did those sorts of things, did not give the extra for the ice-cream, and did not buy the cheese and tomatoes. But why should my mother be criticised for that? Plenty of women manage the housekeeping as she did, but it does not matter because they have enough, more than enough.

Childhood teas with Mother! Once she brought home a long handled spoon from a café – stole it, I suppose. It was the sort you use to eat an ice cream sundae out of a tall glass. But we did not have any glasses like that, so I don't know how we were supposed to benefit from it. Maybe she just liked having a bit of the café at home with her, to remind her.

She usually had her hat on. Or sometimes a comb stuck in her hair. Too restless to finish the combing, just as she was too restless to hold a baby with its bottle.

On more than one occasion, when I was older, I came in from school to be greeted by her holding her hands over her eyes, and telling me not to worry, not to worry, which of course made me worry. I soon saw that the front of her hair was singed, and then that her eyebrows were burnt off. She had turned the gas on and then gone looking for a match!

*

Sorting through yet more of my mother's things, having come back from another visit to Fawsett House with only tea and biscuits this time, the bundles of letters remind me again of the clock on the mantelpiece, which used to topple over sometimes from the stack of papers put behind it. I think again of those childhood tea times, and the memory jogs yet again.

When she was about eight years old, my second daughter, Hayley, came home from having tea with a school friend, and when I asked her what she had been given for tea she told me she had had baked beans and bread. 'With bread?' I asked. 'Not toast?'

'No. Tina made it.'

'Was the mother not there? I asked, alarm bells ringing.

'Oh, yes, her mother was there.'

'What did you have to drink?'

'Water, just a cup of water.' A cup! So they had no drinking glasses either, like us.

Hayley then revealed that Tina's mother had been sitting in an armchair all the time the children made and ate tea. She was drinking cups of tea and listening to the radio. 'She didn't seem to notice us,' my daughter said.

I think of maternal neglect. Like our mother sending us to school dressed without care, a child of five being sent to school with a heavy cold and no hanky. Is it neglect? Or is it something else? I wonder as I fix a few letters with an elastic band and throw some old bills into a carrier bag for my bin. There is little paper rubbish to go through now. I am sorting it with half my mind while the other half thinks of my mother and of mothers in general. Then, my attention is grabbed again when another picture postcard appears, this time showing a pier. I am back, five years ago, on the pier at Worthing with mother.

*

A sheltered division runs the length of the pier, from the entrance, with its restaurant, ice-cream and other shops. Long benches stand at intervals along it, and the day is warm. I am walking towards my mother, who is reading the Daily Mirror, bought near the bus stop in Surbiton, and shading her eyes with her hands. I have been to buy an ice-cream. I see a woman about my mother's age coming towards us from the entrance. She walks on crutches because she only has one leg and, when she reaches us, she asks if there is room for her on the seat.

Mother looks up from her paper and asks the woman what happened to her leg. She is asking the question I did not like to ask. The woman tells us that, whilst out playing with her many brothers and sisters in a rough part of London, she knocked her leg on a rusty iron bar. Her leg hurt for days, and the wound was starting to look increasingly bad. In the end, she was taken to hospital where doctors decided that the only way to save her life was to amputate the leg. They said this would not have happened had she been brought in earlier.

'Why didn't your mother take you to a doctor earlier? I ask.

'I don't think she noticed.'

'Didn't notice you had a bad leg?

'I don't think she noticed anything very much. She had thirteen children.' 'How did you cope? Learn to manage on one I leg, I mean? Did your mother help you?' She laughed, 'I don't think she even noticed I only had one leg.' To manage with one leg for most of your life, I am thinking, and then I ask.

'Did you ever marry?'

'Oh no dear, I've never had anything to do with any man. All they give you is children and no money.' I get up and go to get her an ice-cream.

*

The memories of Worthing fade and I am tired of the sorting. I decide to pamper myself with a long soak in a bubbly bath, and there I try to work out what is the matter with mothers, with my mother in particular. Mothers, who ignore, neglect and damage. I see again my mother running in and out of our table with a knife sticking out. Was it apathy, inertia, resentment, illness? I know when I was about twelve my mother was told she had anaemia, that she must have had it for years and that they had only just caught it in time. Was that due to all the living off scraps off our plates? Had it taken its toll? I wonder. But why deny herself as well as us? Why punish everybody? Or do we all do just that?

Well, I think, topping up the bath with more hot water, most mothers in the past would not have been able to indulge like this. They very often had no bath, and if they did, could not afford to use much hot water. Wrapped in a fluffy towel, given to me for Christmas by Anna and her family, I wipe the steam from the bathroom mirror, and look at my face. I still look good, and yet I am filled with despair and anger that my face has not been my fortune, or even brought me any love. How much longer can my looks last – long enough to meet a man – before they are ruined by so many bad times? I stay in front of the mirror and do some face exercises, then some pelvic muscle squeezing. It is then that I remember that I have been just like Tina's mother, and the one leg lady's mother – and my own.

I recall in the early days of my divorce from my children's father, that my youngest brother Gordon came to see me. Soon after he drove away, he crashed his car into a tree. Somehow, he limped back to knock on my door, his face covered in blood. And I sent him across the road to my friend who was a nurse. Afterwards, he told me that he had been scared to come to me after the accident, because he thought it would be too much of a shock for me

'But it didn`t seem to have much effect on you,' he said.

No, I must admit I felt nothing – it hardly registered what he was saying or what his face looked like. I was in so much trouble inside that I could not take on any more. I had too much pain of my own. I was on overload with misery, and I can remember thinking that night, when he had finally gone home, that was how it must be in war-torn zones. When your first relative is killed you would be distraught, and when the second is killed, the third, the fourth, the fifth, you would be distraught over and over again. But I imagine that there must come a time when you could feel no more. No further death would touch you. Even now, as I wipe out the bath, I do not know whether that is because you are on overload, or because your feelings become numb. Perhaps it is the same thing. What is it with the mother who does not notice the bad leg, the mother who cuts herself off with tea and radio and is unaware that children are making their own beans and bread? Is it lack of money? Too many children? Perhaps lack of glamour? It is certainly lack of anything that makes the hard work of child care bearable, even possible, as in the case of money. Many times in my childhood, my mother told me that she was crying inside.

The knife flashes through my memory again. I was very small, and there was only my first brother and me there, and my mother shook a knife at his throat. She was gripping the handle, and the face and voice frightened me. It was almost the 'gertcha, gertcha' of the pavement and car scene. I did not do or say anything. I guess that, though only three, I had learnt not to be a nuisance and to push any feelings away, perhaps because I was already on overload. Or already had low expectations. Could it be that I already accepted horror as the norm? Sometimes I think that I barely have feelings, but when and how were they stifled?

It is only now that I talk of the incident to my children and to Gordon. I have never mentioned it to Victor. We were not the sort of family who talked about anything serious. Gordon says we were like six strangers living under one roof, and between some of us this state still exists.

For many seconds I watched as my mother held a knife at my brother's throat.

Beautiful Dreamer

Chapter 7

I arrive at Fawsett House to the usual greeting from Mother, about the suitcases, solicitors and being depressed, and why can't she come and stay with me, 'just for a little while.' I feel desperate and weary. My mother's language over the past thirty years has been so clever, 'only for a little while,' or 'just for once.' How I hate those words, `just` and `only.` `Just get me a loaf while you are out shopping,' when 'just' turns out to mean a ten minute queue, and you were not going near the bread shop anyway. 'Can you look after my five children? I'll only be half an hour.' Then the half an hour becomes two hours and the children tear the house apart.

When I took my mother out for a day, she always wanted that extra hour. 'Only for an hour,' she would say. She would then want to come back with me, 'just for a quick cup of tea.' My fear took the form of a growing monster. We would stay out longer, and she would come into my house 'only for a minute,' then would become all pathetic when I said it was time to go home.

Whenever it was the end of an outing, she would become angry and aggressive, asking why I wanted to get rid of her. `Why do you ration me? ` She says it even now, every time I leave Fawsett House. In those days of the regular Sunday car outings, the demands to come home with me at the end of the day were always there to dread. I had terrifying visions of her staying for the evening, then for the night, then forever!

Some people have never tuned in to social convention, the games, the giving somebody the message, the getting the messages oneself. So they ask the embarrassing, awkward and unaskable questions. It has always seemed to me that my mother's indirect question is 'do you love me? And 'why don't you love me? ` Yet behind that, I read that I have to love her, or she will destroy me, maybe kill me. She has almost killed me inside.

We have only a tray of tea things between us on the table today. I pour the tea and watch my mother balance the cup not quite right on the saucer, not in its circular groove. She has always done this, and it has always driven me mad. 'They say I can't manage myself,' she says in a whisper, and I try to think of how I can tell her that she can't. I remember some years back when she made a foul mess in the toilet of a pub. I couldn't cope. We just left. I could not face cleaning it myself, and could not face the pub people..

I am about to explain, but I get out of it because she is busy with her tea and choosing biscuits, so I look around at the lolling heads. Do they sleep away whatever time is left to them because to be conscious is to be in hell? Have they had neither fulfilment nor joy? If not, they will hardly expect any now. Has it all been so hard and nobody knows? All anybody knows is that they were 'bad mothers'? Or does the worst pain come from everyone telling them they have nothing to complain about?

One beauty had been awakened by visitors today, and there is a new baby in the family, dressed in blue. The granddaughter holds her baby close to her grandmother, and the baby screams. Is that through revulsion at the lined and sunken face, and the awareness that this is the baby's destiny? Or is it because he can sense the old age rejection of him? I have sensed no joy in my mother at the arrival of her great grandchildren. Resentment seemed more apparent than that, and I have understood that what I see is jealousy at the great fuss made about babies. Who makes a fuss of her?

Yet they must have done once, for most babies get some welcome and many a lot more than that. But it ends. It must do for people to live such troubled lives, for people to reach the end of their lives as wretched as my mother is, as wretched as most of these residents look. Does it end when the baby no longer looks cute, or when its interests conflict with yours? Whenever I hear of a man convicted of murder, I think how once he was a newborn baby, with so much promise.

A lot of old people are not cared for. A lot of people much younger are not cared for. Yet if a baby is shown time and attention and consideration, why does not everybody get that throughout life, for they are only the baby grown older? If the old are abandoned, why, when they were once that adorable baby? If anyone matters at all then everyone does. We are at any stage part of the same continuum.

The woman in the winter coat and thick socks walks in. 'She never stops walking,' says Mother, watching the woman go over to the baby and stop walking long enough to look.

'Why do you wear your coat on such a lovely day? Asks the young mother, we are well into autumn now, but today it is like an Indian summer.

'What's it to do with you? If I were too hot, I would take it off, wouldn't I?` I have never heard the walker speak before, and her voice is as harsh and as rasping as are my feelings looking at her poor mottled legs. She leaves the room and walks out into the entrance hall. It is time for me to leave too. I glance at my watch and Mother does not miss it.

'You are always looking at your watch when you are with me,' she complains. 'Why do you ration me?'

'I am going swimming,' I say, and get up to go. As I kiss my mother goodbye, I think of the picture I have seen of her as a young child. She had a pert little face with a pointed chin, thick curly auburn hair, and of course the big bow. Yet now, that little girl's daughter does not want to be with her more than duty demands, there is nothing about her which brings pleasure.

I walk to the main door, ready to press the code which will allow me to leave, but the walker is there first and is opening the door. I know that she sometimes goes for a walk or even to the corner shop to buy sweets, newspapers, and anything else the residents ask for. 'Where are you going?` I ask.

'None of your business,' she snaps. 'How rude.' The rough, gruff voice is almost masculine, like the cropped hair and the grizzled head.

As I search for my car keys, I see Ann Wright approaching the door I have left. She was my mother's Social Worker when she lived in her own home, and still liaises with the home on client care. She has always called my mother's state 'anxiety' and I have not been able to find the words I want to say: 'anxious about what? ` I feel there is so much more to my mother than just that. I walk back and speak to her. After a quick recap on my mother's settling into the home, I ask her about the residents and why they sleep so much. She says it is because they are weary, and weary of what, I think. I can hardly share with her my half-formed theories that they sleep to escape the lack of their past and the hopelessness of their future. I ask if they all get visitors and she confirms that many get none at all. In her job she meets with the cases we all hear about, the old person found in their home, dead for many days and with nobody knowing.

'But in my experience,' she says, 'that never happens except where they have been a bad parent.' I am about to ask how she knows that and what does she mean by 'bad,' when suddenly she looks thoughtful and adds, 'sometimes, though, there has been poverty that the children never knew about.' And other lacks they were unaware of too, I think.

That night, in my sleep, I have a vision. My mother and I are setting a table together. I do not like it. As I wake, I know it is a vision that, in some way off time, somewhere, in another world perhaps, my mother and I will be together as equal women, equal providers, carers and caterers. There is something I do not like about this idea of my mother seen to be an equal carer with me, my history with her forgotten, as though it had never been. I suppose my complaint is similar to that of the brother of the Prodigal son, for we are not equal carers and providers right now. I sometimes feel like the unpaid carer of the universe.

I don't think it would make up for it all now, if she brought me tea on a saucer with care. I don't know if I could bear it now.

The vision, dream, or whatever it was, disturbs and hurts me. I suppose because my mother's 'vision' of my true destiny is that of carer; and hers the one I care for. I carry within me a silent raging anger that, not in her opinion or desires, but as a truth, I am on this earth to be her provider, that I really AM her mother, sister, husband, lady's maid, cosy aunt and buddy, buddy friend. Funny how these ideas of someone's role spreads out to others. I have felt with many people in my life that I am seen as an all providing, plastic, mamma!

She believes I am those roles, but a failure in them all. I cannot cope with what she thinks I am, a cosy home body, and that all my forays into Adult Education, and even a degree, are just me messing about and rebelling. My mother will never see me as clever. I 'just work hard.'

She creates the picture by cutting off the bits of the negative she does not like. She does not know what degree I got, and does not even listen when I tell her I have had a short story published. These facts do not fit in with her chosen reality.

Back in time again and it is Christmas, I am twenty-four years old and have a small child and new baby. My husband has bought me a short skirt and a skinny rib sweater for Christmas, and we all gather at the house of my older brother with my parents. Mother looks at my clothes. 'He wants you to be a modern girl, some 'kookie' or something. You are not. You are a sweet, kind, gentle cosy....' Her view of me, her view of my husband's view of me – my husband's actual view of me – where was the real me in all this?

Basically, she destroyed any sense of worth I might have had because her message was clear, that I had no needs, was only here to fulfil the needs of others. If my sister broke my doll when I was at school and she was under school age, it was simply that I should have let her have my doll anyway. And so from a very early age I was the family victim and so became a possible victim for others. I had one abusive relationship after another, each one worse than the one before, until the last one, which almost destroyed me. I was left so emotionally and financially depleted that I ended up living in my last choice area, round the corner from my mother. I read my spiritual and psychology books all the time. Reading of the power of the mind, I came to believe that her strong intent created the circumstances she wanted, me on her doorstep, free to dance attendance on her.

'Why do you ration me? The first time this was said was a few years ago now. `You used to see me more often, in the sixties when the girls were small. You seemed to be more happy-go-lucky then.'

`But I wasn't happy in those days,' I replied.

`Oh, I know you weren't happy,' she said. ' I was. I was enjoying myself.' I wondered if what she was actually saying was that she was enjoying having me on a piece of string. get nowhere if I try to discuss the way she treats me. If I complain about something she has said or done, she denies it, or says she was only trying to help and advise. If I then press further, with more detailed examples, she says, 'well, that is only a small thing.' When nearly cornered, she resorts to reminding me that I allow this person or that person to do the same to me, and when she can no longer think of anything to say, I get, 'Oh you do go on so.'

There is a complete disregard for me, even strangers come first. Once, I was in a restaurant with her and I was smoking. The person on the next table was fanning the smoke with their hands, and glowering at me, despite the fact that we were in a 'smoking 'section of the restaurant. Mother told me that I should stop because I was upsetting them.

I have always taken her to parks and riversides, and she has always complained that we do not spend longer there. I am agoraphobic, and in those places, I often feel lost, bleak, frightened, or peculiar. In the early years of this condition, after my second child was born, even a trip to the local shops could bring on a panic attack, I just had to get home. All mother said at the time was that my husband had brain washed me so that he would not have to take me out! Now, she says that maybe I will come to love one day the places she adores. If the person in my vision is my mother one wondrous day, what of how it is for me now? Is it all to be wiped out? These thoughts have been filling my head during my twenty minute meditation – Transcendental Meditation does allow thoughts to drift in. What can I do to make Mother treat me differently? What can I do to bring her some happiness? What of my greater happiness? Transcending through meditation is supposed to manifest all good things into your life. After the meditation I allow myself two squares of chocolate.

Chapter 8

'I can't begin to tell you ...' Mother greets me on my next visit to the Home. She speaks like a duchess who is about to tell you about the problems she is having with the servants. Mother has her best voice on today, almost 'posh', but she is acting, and she speaks as though what she is about to tell me is interesting, important or deep. It turns out that what she can't begin to tell me is how depressed she is, as if this were some amazing new revelation. Mother used to speak like this when she arrived at my house and would start berating me about some member of the family, then go on to criticise me for my dress, my home, my children, in fact my whole way of life. Oh, and of course my hair, especially my hair. Somehow the 'posh' voice gave her the sound of authority, but it was all an act. I knew that, I had observed the exact same scenario many times before.

I sit and listen to the endless babble, my mind elsewhere. This change of voice has evoked another memory, and I am back to the time when I was reading for my degree at a local University. I had not seen my mother for a while as I still had all the children at home, and it was difficult enough to fit everything in. Mother had been ill with shingles, and I had not been able to visit her. Now, she was well enough for an outing to the Spiritualist Church and had telephoned me to say that if she could get herself on the bus to my college, would I drive her the two towns away to the church in Hampton Hill. Of course, my conscience had to say yes. I came out of my lecture to find her in the entrance hall, on a chair, apparently asleep, her head lolled, her mouth open, and she looked dreadful. In fact, my initial reaction was that she looked more 'dead' than asleep. I had already been treated to weeks of telephone calls about how wretched it is to be ill when you live on your own; for, as I had been unable to visit, she had remained unvisited and in her mind that meant unloved. Nobody to bring her a cup of tea in bed when she was ill she kept saying. I had failed in my role of the little girl carrying tea to her mother with such care – failed yet again.

I approached this dead-looking figure full of guilt, remembering what my father said when I was six, that if Mum died it would be my fault. Having discovered her to be alive after all, I rushed off to get my car, which was parked a few streets away. I was extremely tired, had an essay to plan and children to feed later –

and really could not spare this time. As I drove back to the college I thought of all the events I had missed out on because I had promised to meet Mother for coffee in Kingston between lectures, all the missed chances of networking with fellow students, and free glasses of wine. As I drove her to the church I saw the 'dead' act for what it was. In my car she was full of life, animated, and ranting nonstop about my busy household, my children, my man friend, and my neighbours' continual visits.

'Are they all still running in and out of the house?'

I knew what was behind all this; she was saying 'I am jealous of your busy life. I want to rub it in, how downtrodden you are, how used by so many people, I want you to give all your time to me, not to them, and I want to be the one who runs in and out of your house.' On and on she went, nag, nag, nag, until I screamed. 'Look, I'm taking you,' I yelled. 'I won't take you if you don't shut up!' She had made me so angry, which is her triumph. I detected a satisfied smirk on her face. She had succeeded.

Then, how had she managed this, I wondered? I thought I was the hired transport only, but the next thing I knew I was sitting inside the church and ended up sitting through the whole service, whilst my children were at home, waiting, alone without me. I had become an accessory, a thing to drive her, a thing to accompany her, a thing to show off – look how my daughter loves me – but on many occasions when I have accompanied her, she has completely ignored me, once she has found someone else to talk to. Was she truly as ill as she looked when I met her at the college? Am I unkind?

She was certainly pushing my buttons yet again.

As I sat, not particularly interested in the service, I remembered another scene. I was about fourteen at the time and her youngest brother Albert was coming to visit. She had a broom in her hand, and was wearing a 'houseworky ' overall. I heard Albert arrive and come through the shop. My mother must surely have heard him too, but she stood, holding the broom, with her back to the kitchen door. As her brother pushed open the door to our kitchen, she did not change her position other than to turn her head and look over her shoulder. What he would have seen is what I saw as I moved near the door to greet him - a face turned to look over the shoulder, the back view of his sister who is so busy she has to be still sweeping when her brother arrives. Even at that young age, I could see the Cinderella act, and recognized the look of mournful pleading on the doleful face. It said it all: 'Look at me, look at the wretched life your poor sister has. Why don't you give me lots of money s I can get away from all this drudgery?'

We children have often wondered whether our dirty, scruffy appearance was all an act too, a sort of cry for help. 'Look how I can't manage my children. Look what a state I am in. Somebody please come and help me.' Yet, I also believe that sometimes the only way we human beings can show our feelings is to 'act' them, because we have become out of the habit of accessing and expressing pain. I am still trying to find what her pain was, and still hope that, somehow, I can take her on holiday before it is too late. I am still dreaming that
she may meet her Prince in the Home.

Beautiful Dreamer

Chapter 9

On my next visit to Fawsett House I am greeted with something completely new. 'Someone's getting into my room.'

Mother explains that she believes that someone is getting into her bedroom and taking her things. She can't find half her clothes, and she still wants her suitcases. She is adamant that someone is in her room when she is downstairs, taking her clothes and putting other women's clothes in her cupboard. The dress she is wearing, she claims, is not hers. She could be right. I was meant to label all her clothes, but have not got round to it. The Carers said they would do it for me, but maybe they are too busy.

Mother is outraged. She does not know what is going on in this place, this dreadful place where I have dumped her. She wants me to bring her a new compact of foundation powder the next time I come, because somebody has stolen the one she had. The dress she is wearing is flowery and reminds me of 'the dress' she wore all the time in the forties. She looks so thin and flat, like an old doll with half the sawdust leaked out through a hole. She was always scrawny when we were children, hardly eating anything except for the bits off our plates and the shop cakes. Then, after my dad died, she got fatter and fatter. Maybe it was through comfort eating when she found that she was all alone. Or maybe she was more contented then and could eat in a way she could not when swamped with the needs of a husband and children?

When our father died, Victor was working abroad as a Ship's Photographer, Gordon was at University, and my sister and I were married, so she had only herself to please. Or maybe the eating was just relief after living for two years with Dad's lung cancer. Since becoming eighty, the weight has been dropping off her. To reveal the perfect figure? Is it her last bid for love? Her last chance to attract the prince who will carry her off from all she does not like, as she hoped her brother would take her from the housework? Or carry her to the dreams which have never come true?

A fatter lady resident joins us at our table with the coffee cups, and looks across at Mother, cupping her own stomach in her hands. 'So you've dropped yours,' she says, pointing to my mother's middle, then adds, 'I have not dropped mine yet.'

She laughs. 'My hubby's been dead for thirty years now.'

I find this remark interesting, and recall when my sister and I, not long married, visited our mother together one day. She stood before us, touching herself all over as she always did, smoothing her hands over her curves and touching her hair, turning her head from side to side. 'There... there hasn't... you know... There hasn't been anything... For four years.' Older women are assumed by many to be asexual, to have forgotten all about it, but here we have the woman of ninety remarking that she could not be pregnant because her husband is dead. We have the woman of fifty-four telling her daughters that sex has ended between her and her husband. What made her mention this? Was it relief, I wonder, or did she miss it? Her seemingly lack of enthusiasm for sex – well abhorrence surely calling it, `that nasty business` – was that caused by having a low sex drive, or because it only brought babies, drudgery and poverty? Would it have been different with a man who had taken her round the world in a camper van, and shown her the attention of a mother, of the bow-tying variety?

With Mother in the Home, I have more time to think, so am trying hard to piece together just what this complicated woman is all about. I remember her past, particularly her past with me, and my focus has been drawn to her sexuality. It came about because of what the nurse said, and in that instant I saw a vision of my mother as a possible 'Sleeping Beauty.'

I know that my dad experienced jealousy about her. She told me when I was still a child that if he saw her talking to a male neighbour in the street, he would come running over to their side, looking full of anger and panic. If she were sexually attractive to men, would that necessarily mean she was interested herself? She told me once that there had been a boy who was in love with her years before she met my dad. He adored her and would sit looking at her with big, pleading eyes, but my mother refused his attentions and offerings of marriage, because she thought that she would end up like the poor wives in aprons. The boy retreated, but she heard later that he pined for ten years, and she thinks he may even have died.

I will never understand why my mother thought marriage meant the apron, the pub, and the ` `is paper' of the young wives who lived near her mother's shop, when she had so many happy, affluent, married relatives. What had happened to make her feel like this? Would it have been different if she had married a man who could give her the gypsy caravan in the form of a camper van?

*

Now I see a series of visions of my parents, flashing across my memory screen one by one. The first is of them meeting at the funfair. I see her big bosom in the Kaiser Bondar brassiere, and the head-turning titian hair flowing in the breeze. I then see them a few years later on holiday with my brother, myself, and my sister who was only a year old. The people in the guest house, the landlady, and the other guests are admiring the baby and saying how lovely she is. My parents lean together and smile like shy children who are not used to praise. Do I see some kind of sexual bond here? For surely my sister was produced through a sexual act. But no, I think it is more likely that the flush of pleasure is that of two uncared for little children, surprised at receiving any kind of acknowledgement or admiration, rather than any sweetness or sexual bond.

In another scene, I see my father in his last days. They are both in their fifties. He is in hospital and my mother is visiting. She looks 'baggy and draggy' these days, always wearing clothes that did not show her shape – and I did not know if she still wore 'the dress' under her outer clothes – but she is carrying a shopping bag, always a shopping bag. When my dad did finally acquire a car, he took her out on Sunday afternoons, when he did not have to work in the shop. They would drive into the country and find somewhere pretty to stop for tea, but Mother always took a shopping bag, as well as her handbag, in case she saw something to buy on the way, some country produce, like eggs.

What must his feelings have been? Here was a dying man, and I know now that he knew it, with his wife bundling towards him carrying the bag. I wonder if he remembered the beauty he had met at the fair? Did he look at this woman, in her fifties, still with a pretty face, but nevertheless a bag lady with a dejected walk and dispirited air? Did he think, 'I have done this to her`? Could there have been, in spite of the years of misery, the 'nasty business,' and no sex, an affection that had grown from familiarity and shared children, at the end? But Mother did tell me, in his last years, that Dad would not let her talk about the children. She said it was cruel, and so it was, but my heart bled for both of them. In, fact, wasn't he being a bit of a Rumpelstiltskin, separating her from her children if only in conversation?

Yet another scene flashes up on my inner slide show now.

It is years after the 'pretty baby' memory of my parents and before the scene which tears my heart, when the dying man was visited by his 'Beauty' turned death-in-life hag. It is of me at my school desk, and my A level class teacher is reading a poem about a wedding cake. On top of the wedding cake stands a model of a bride and his groom. They represent the parents of the poet. The little man doll bows to his bride and the tears fall down my cheeks. For I knew it was not like that for my parents, and my father had never revered his wife.

I remember now, sitting with my mother in a park when my father had been dead for seven years. Another older lady joined us and asked my mother how long she has been a widow. 'Oh about five years, I think,' said Mother. I can remember thinking how sad that she hadn't been counting the years.

The last scene to flick on my memory screen is of my father's funeral. My mother has chosen roses, and I can see them on top of the coffin. My mother walks behind the coffin and, turning into the chapel, one red rose is suddenly blown off the wreath by the wind. It lands at her feet. Surely this was a message from dad, from the heavens, that he wanted, at last, to give her honour due?

Chapter 10

'Where are my shoes?' This is the greeting from my mother today as I visit. She is wearing her slippers, like the other residents, who wear them most of the time. 'I can't go out without my shoes,' Mother complains, and I distract her with the sweets I have bought her as well as the new compact. I notice she is now much frailer, and apart from resenting the time and the energy needed to take her out, I do not have the courage.

The lady who has not yet 'dropped hers' is wearing a cardigan, and I think of my 'Cardigan Girl.' Does she wear her woolly jacket in the same way as my mother wore 'the dress,' as a kind of message that she does not want sex? The old ladies' cardigan is pulled across what at first looks like a flat chest; in fact it looks like only skin where the bulge should be, and the what is really the bulge of them balloons down near the waist.

'Shall I bring my mother in some bras? I ask the Carer, 'it looks uncomfortable like that.'

'They don't seem to bother about them,' the Carer explains.

'They have their vests, they all like their vests.' Do vests give them support, I wonder, or is the vest like 'the dress'? I look more closely at my mother, and it is as though her breasts are a pair of tights, hung up Christmas Eve night, and in the morning they still hang, like a string, with an orange in each toe. What of the 'perfect figure' the nurse described? Maybe she meant the in-and-out of the waist and hips, or maybe because she dealt with my mother in a lying down position, so the breasts were not hanging?

I recall when I first noticed my mother's body and think they were not much better then. Our parents were late getting up on one of Dad's rare Sundays off, and one by one we drifted into their room. Her nightdress was open at the front, and we could see these flat hanging things. I remember I played with her travelling bag, like a box shaped cosmetic one, but firmer like a suitcase, and with a zip all around it. It contained brushes for hair, clothes, and shoes, as well as a mirror, comb, and nail file. She told me it was meant for holidays. I wonder who gave it to her, or whether she brought it for herself.

Did she ever use that travelling kit, I wonder? But if she
had, would it have made any difference to her inner world? She
once escaped for a few days to Worthing, but was lonely in the
evenings. Oh, how I have dreamed that, on one of those
evenings, she danced off to the pier, and met the man who had
been pining for her so long. I think of those sad lonely evenings
alone in Worthing, and recall another sad painful loneliness for
me.

It was on a holiday, when we went as a family to a Butlin's
holiday camp. Mother had suffered one of her then frequent
asthma attacks. It haunted me for years, but I'd forgotten about it
up until now. She told me, when I was still young, how she had
sat outside our holiday chalet all night – alone – and unable to
breathe.

I suddenly remember that Mother once told me her early life
was ruined by hay fever. Sad for someone who so wanted to be
outside.

Thoughts of Worthing bring me back to the present and remind
me that I have forgotten to give her the second postcard, the one
showing the pier. I rummage through my handbag and show it to
her. 'Oh yes, my Worthing,' she says.
'Will you take me there? They don't seem to arrange any outings
in this Day Centre. Will you take me there soon?' And what are
we going to do when we get there, I think to myself, other than
elevenses, lunch and tea? She always likes my company, wants
my company, and needs my company, but is no company to me.

'Why can't you give me a bit of your time? she is always saying.
'You never have time for a quiet talk these days.' What do we
ever talk about Mother? Other than how terrible the world is, and
how selfish or nasty most of our relatives are? The government
has taken away half your buses and most of your public seats, or
the foreigners take what seats there are, and that I should give
you more of my time, and I really ought to have you to live with
me, since you are no trouble. And my hair is a mess and do I
want to borrow your comb.

The walking lady, who wears her coat indoors as well as out,
passes, then goes out through the French windows. There are
plants at the side of these windows, in fact there are plants all
around the Home, and some have gnomes sitting in them. There

are also large print books, and even a few toys to entertain visiting children. I think of the plants and how planting into a larger pot will make them grow bigger. Would my mother have grown if she had travelled – been in a larger pot of the world? Or is the size of the pot nothing to do with physical space, but to do with inner horizons, starting with the seed itself?

Mother's conversations have always been very limited, the government, the foreigners, my failure and neglect. On all subjects Mother has a limited repertoire. For example, she says she is 'a cut above the rest,' and has cultural interests like music and history, but when asked what music she likes, she answers, 'nice music.' Pop music she has always detested, the exception being the songs of the Beatles when they first came on the scene, but she hated the 'dreary old Beethoven,' my father played upstairs while she did her pools in the kitchen. When you press further what music she likes, she will say Puccini, and even further, Madam Butterfly, and if you probe on it is always the one aria, 'One Fine Day.' She supposedly 'knows all about history' too, but questioning will only bring Henry VIII, and when asked what she knows about that particular king, she can only talk of him chopping off his wives` heads.

She picks up her new compact now as she rehearses her new lines. Somebody pinched her other compact. People get into her room and take things. She is not joining any more Day Centres, they are all the same. She did not ask to come here. They can't keep her here, and she is going to sue someone, and I must take her out of here, take her home with me.

'Who got me in here? It was you, wasn't it?'

'No Mum, it was the doctors and your Social Worker.'

'Then I'll sue them. I never did like that Social Worker. I'm going to change her.'

'But you would not want to be in that flat Mum. They took you back there, remember, you said you did not want to live there anymore.'

'No, I was with Mum just before I came here.'

This is a new one.

'Why can't I go back and live with my mum?'

'Your mother died nearly fifty years ago.' I try to sound gentle.

'She can't have done.' She is quiet now and looks puzzled.

'But I remember. I was with Mum just before I came here.'

'You're just remembering some other time, Mum,' I try again.

'No, I was with Mum. She was putting my coat on me.'
wonder where she was going, where she was been sent, that time that her mum was putting her coat on little Nellie. Was her mum brushing her hair, and tying on the brown velvet bow too? Why does she want to go back to Mum and the shop?

'Were you happy, at home? I ask, hoping for something new.

'Well, Mum did her best. She broke her arm, you see.' We are back to the old repertoire. I wonder about the limits of her experience. It is as though she has stayed in a very small pot. Or is she blocking out something in her past? She has lived a long life, with thirty years behind the shop, thirty years as wife and mother, then thirty years of widowhood. Yet she has narrowed down her long life to being a small child behind the shop with Mum. It is as though the rest did not happen, and she was with her mum yesterday.

Chapter 11

Mother used to steal lipsticks.

I can see her now coming to my home from the shops. suppose to her I am one of the poor wives and cannot afford many lipsticks, and it is perfectly all right, because what she steals is the samples. They are the lipsticks that stick out from the display full of lipstick shaped holes, for women to try the colour on their wrists. Unlike the ones you buy, they have no lids, and at the end is a 'sticking-out bit,' which is lipstick shaped and shows the colour so you know which one to try.

This made them difficult to use, especially when putting them on in public. I had to try and hide the sticking out bit in the palm of my hand, until my sister told me that you could break it off, and that bit in itself, Valerie and I discovered, was full of lipstick which you can get out with the aid of a lip brush.

The only trouble is that Mother's 'pinching' means fewer lipsticks for customers to use as samples. Others must take them too, for these racks are often depleted. One of my neighbours amused me when she came in from a trip to Kingston, and an abortive search for a lipstick in the colour she wanted, and said to me, ` I think your mother must have been at the lipstick counter again.'

When my mother visited me in my young motherhood days, she would always bring broken biscuits, special-offer grocery items, jumble sale children's clothes, and sometimes stolen lipsticks. I never used the jumble clothes. We were brought up in them and Mother wears them still. She brought me dresses for my newborn first baby, and I used them for dusters. I could not bring myself to put them on my baby girl, even though we sometimes did not have enough clothes for her to keep up with the washing.

Once my mother's last baby was out of nappies, she cut them into strips and used them as sanitary towels. Whether she then washed them or threw them away, I do not know. When I began periods she was angry that she had to buy me 'things,' and when the woman in the shop showed my mother the range of sanitary belts, she said I could pin the towels to my vest. I wonder at the self abasement of so many women. I have seen women wear rags to send their child to a private school. I knew a woman who fed her children, not eating herself, but telling them she had eaten earlier when she had not. My mother ate the scraps off our plates.

Is wearing jumble sale clothes and using rags as sanitary protection some kind of self-punishment? If so, why? Is it the guilt of being female? The guilt, which I have heard was once in women, of being `dirty` in producing babies out of your body? My mother once said that she realised a woman should keep herself clean and not allow herself to get pregnant, but when I asked her what she meant, she described in a roundabout way some kind of post coital douching. After she had me, she went through the Church of England's service of 'Churching,' a form of thanksgiving for the safe-delivery of a baby, and the survival of the mother, but it is also a ritual of cleansing. It was only the cleansing purpose of the service that my mother knew about, and she thought that it was a very nice idea.

Yet, as well as treating herself shabbily like this, in other areas she was lavish in taking at least small treats. She spent money on the pictures, and ate cream cakes in cafés.

She went to jumble sales and parks, when she could have been cleaning the house or washing our clothes. She frittered money on her jaunts so that there was little left over for new clothes, or sanitary towels, and certainly nothing for little bits and pieces to brighten up the home.

Our family income was indeed very low, especially for four children, and I doubt whether less gallivanting and frittering would have made much of a difference. If we had been the kind of family who had clean table cloths and a cake making mother, we might also have been the family to spend money on visiting distant relations, entertaining them to Sunday dinner, or even putting money in a church collection. But I find the contrast of denying herself, and the indulgences, an interesting parallel compared with the way she could be so rebellious, yet so submissive too.

Chapter 12

'They tell me I can go home any time I like.' This is Mother's greeting today. 'When I ask them if I can go, they say, 'Ask you daughter, ask Patricia.' Then she adds, 'do you want to borrow my comb? She looks pityingly at my hair, and begins rummaging in her handbag, fortunately getting sidetracked from the comb as she comes upon her compact. Mother looks in the compact's little mirror, and puts the foundation powder and cream onto her nose and cheeks. I remember women's make-up when I was a child, and how Mother and the mothers of friends dabbed their noses with powder and put lipstick on, but I cannot recall ever seeing them use eye makeup. I do remember something called rouge, which was a redder or deeper pink powder which some women put on their cheeks, making them look like painted dolls.

It never ceases to delight and amaze, these lifelong desires in women to look good. Once upon a time, I read of a woman who was held as a prisoner of war. Every day, she kept back her portion of margarine from her ration of food to use on her face, to prevent her skin from becoming dry and chapped. In these days I have been told that many starving women in the world will dye their lips and put on beads so they look good.

I look across the tea cups, yet again, at my mother with the flowered dress pulled across the completely flat chest. It physically pains me to see the breast tissue hanging by the waist. She is wearing her golden cross, and is showing it to me yet again, since for a few weeks she had mislaid it, and had been sure it was 'stolen' from her room. The cross is beautiful, and is real gold, given to her one Christmas by my daughter, Hayley. Mother is obviously very proud of it, as she is of any gift that looks expensive, I think to myself. Sometimes she does get it a bit wrong, the way she assesses the value of something, judging a birthday card by its size, when it might be cheap and tacky. For example a 'Dearest Mum' card, with sparkly bits on it, delights her, while she hardly looks at the expensive, art design one which is smaller.

I look around the room at my 'Sleeping Beauties' and notice that they are all wearing necklaces and brooches, my mother is wearing a brooch today, which I don't remember, so I ask her where she got it. 'That nice lady over there gave it to me,' she says, indicating the one who 'has not dropped hers,' but whose hubby has been dead for thirty years.

'Did she not want it? I ask.

'She said she has too many brooches, and she'd noticed I never wore one.' A little bit of girly fun, I wonder, giving, sharing, and swapping?

The moustache lady comes in, walking her mother-in-law slowly into the large conservatory where I sit with Mother. She joins us and the two older ladies begin to talk, so I talk to the 'moustache lady.' She tells me yet again how her husband died suddenly and how his mother swiftly began to decline, bringing her into Fawsett House. Is that it, I wonder?
Is senility one way of escaping insufferable pain? If you cannot bear the loss of a son, do you push it away and act as if you don't know? You will be seen as mad, yes, but that seeming madness is perhaps your way of creating a reality that is more bearable than the real one.

As the daughter-in-law talks to me, I wonder again if letting her appearance go is a way of avoiding hurt. She is younger than I am and could well meet a new partner, have a new life. But if she allows herself to look totally unattractive, then she will not be seen to be looking, or hoping, and will not therefore be seen to fail. On the other hand, maybe she does not know what to do about her moustache, or cannot afford to do anything about it. She should not have to face that as well as all her other problems of widowhood, and a senile mother-in-law.

How cruel is nature I think to myself. The hormones which attract with their blossom and bloom when you are young, sometimes trapping you into a wrong marriage or too soon motherhood, are the same hormones that produce the wrinkled skin and hairy face which means you can kiss goodbye to any sexual dreams, because nobody will want to kiss you.

The four of us sit together and both older ladies discuss the hairdresser. She has visited Fawsett House today and all the ladies have soft fluffy hair. My mother's hair is the thickest here. She still has the glorious thickness that her mother loved to brush, and it even has just one remnant of a tinge left, on the front wisp, a pale vestige of the auburn colour. (Gasping to stay alive?) Her skin is perfect too, and in fact she is still pretty. True, she does suffer from facial hair, but she also has it removed whenever she can. But is she pretty enough for a lover, even one her age, I ask myself.

'She is a good hairdresser,' my mother is saying. 'You ought to go to her.' She turns to me. 'She'd do your hair a lot better.' She, who stole lipsticks and bled into rags, now abases me. I tell my mother I am leaving and she speaks again, bullying me about giving her more of my time, although the 'moustache lady' left ten minutes ago. The mother-in-law tells me her son is coming soon, and wanders off.

I ask Mother when did Victor, Gordon or Valerie, last visit. She growls at me. ` Don't you go on about the others.`

I put on my coat and explain that I am going swimming. I must get to the pool before four in order to use my cheap ticket for people on benefit. 'Then you should have come earlier,' Mother snaps at my retreating back.

Relieved to be out of the confines of Fawsett House, I pay my fee and walk down the stairs at the swimming baths, undress, and place my things in the locker. I hold onto the rail as I lower myself gently down the pool's steps and into the cold water. I am always cold, due to my circulation, but sometimes I wonder if it never got going because my body – my whole system – was never warmed by a welcoming mother.

Up and down the pool I go, counting the lengths to twenty. Then there is the reverse of up the steps, shower, take things out of the locker, dry and dress, upstairs and out into the world outside. I look at my hair in the mirror of the changing area. It is wet as I never wear a swimming hat. The children's father once told me that he had to wear a hat for an underwater swimming club he joined. It was divided into segments, red and yellow, and he said he looked like a beach ball. It is true that he had a very round face, and I do not, but it always seems to me that mine is large, and that I would look silly – like a beach ball too.

There is nothing I can do here about my hair. It is wet, short and flat. The hairdressers these days are insisting that I must wear it short, 'because long hair drags your face down as you get older,' and they have created a style that is supposed to stick up on top to give me more shape. But my hair never looks, after I have done it myself, as it does when I leave the salon. They blow dry and wax the top into fashionable spikes, which just flop for me.

It is all a chore, like this swimming, but I do that to keep fit. I do it to counteract the effects of a lifetime of abuse. Beginning with a mother who created in me a complete sense of having no rights, I have gone from one abusive relationship to another. I know it all began with Mother when she condoned my sister for breaking my toys. Then, when I was eight years old she told me that I had to 'think of other people.' Consequently I have always put everyone first, never wanted to upset, only wanting to please.

'Don't go on about the others,' she has just said to me. Sometimes I have tried to delegate her care, and she has told me off for 'worrying the others.' Once she said to me, 'how would you like it if I telephoned your son and told him his mother needed help?'

'It's not the same,' I protested.

'Why isn't it? She genuinely sounded confused, and I was not able to explain that my son was not dumping his responsibility on her – it would not have been a case of her delegating as I was trying to do. Sometimes I do not answer because I am tongue-tied, or scared, but at other times – and this was one – I cannot identify exactly what I want to say.

There have been many moments in my life when it would have made an enormous difference if I could have answered what was said to me, but somehow I have always been tongue-tied. Was it because I had been programmed early to 'think of others' and that I did not count?

Not that I blame my siblings for their lack of help. Mother is not an easy person to be with and, briefly, drives everyone mad. If you have her for Sunday lunch, or take her out for the day, it is always complaints about the food or whatever the entertainment, attacks on your way of life or your spouse, or your children, moans about everything from her flat to the lack of buses and seats everywhere, and always the moan that the outing is not long enough and when can she do it again. You end up exhausted. None of us has ever been able to explain it to anyone else, but you will end up with your brain feeling as if it has been scrambled. Why do I stick it? Is it out of pity? Or out of duty? Or in the hope that she will improve, or that one day she will see me differently? Will perhaps one day even like me? Of course there is the guilt loaded on my head by my father. When I did my degree there was no praise from my mother. When other people gave me that in her hearing she would say, 'the only thing is, it meant she saw less of me.'

On my way home from swimming, I called on Anna and her children. Gregory is there as well as Molly, Anna's young daughter. Gregory is a big boy now and mostly walks to and from school, when I look after them. I tell the children now about my hair, and how I can't get the spikes to stay up.

'Try twisting them,' Gregory says. 'When you are blow drying, twist the hair. Hold it upwards and twist it.' This intrigues me, and I drive home thinking how funny to be given hair advice from your grandson, and decide to write a magazine story about it.

Back in the house, I hang up my wet costume and towel. Well, that is over for now, but even as I do length number twenty, I know that it will all start again in a few days time. I exercise regularly, aware that I am possibly saving my life.
For I have read those lists in magazines of the stress points earned by certain life events: death, divorce, moving house, loss of job and the new one which is the leaving of home by adult children. One list told me that if you have too many of these factors, you will add up a total of stress points which could well lead to serious illness

I really do not enjoy swimming and wish I could find something else to do, but exercise classes are beyond my budget. I have lost assets, income, my home area, and the last two years of my younger children being at home, and I have been unable to find work. At first I looked for work and was on Jobseekers' Allowance, but for the last two years, I have been signed off sick with stress and depression.

I walk down to the kitchen where I begin making a stew of soya and root vegetables. I look at the kitchen, it needs decorating, needs all its fixtures replacing, but there is nothing I can do. I don't even like the house. It was all I could get after the debacle, and it screams destruction to me. It screams, `Mug, for allowing yourself to be so trounced.`

Tonight, I have a Marmite pot to wash out into my stew. hate to waste anything and wash out jars into my dinner whenever they are nearly empty, pickle, jam, marmalade, tomato sauce, mustard, anything.

At least I do not have to telephone Mother, I think as I sit on my bed to eat my meal. When she lived in her flat, I phoned her every evening at six. That is over, and at this moment I make up my mind to visit the Home only once a week instead of two. Mother will not notice. Her mind has deteriorated and she has lost all sense of time, believing that she has been in the `Day Centre` as she calls it for only two weeks. Well, that is handy for me. In fact, she has been at Fawsett House for six months, and it is nearly Christmas. Oh, how it rankled me every Christmas before she went into the Home, how the tension mounted as the occasion approached. She always went to Victor for the holiday period, and always gave me the dig about having been going there for so many years. 'He's had me for fourteen years now,' she would gloat.

'I have you every weekend,' I managed to say, on the one occasion when I had not been tongue-tied.

'What do you do? You only take me out once a week.' The word 'only' again, it stabbed at me. Apart from the Sunday drive, I manage most of her affairs, filling in her forms, liaising with doctors and Social Workers, organizing her incontinence pads, obtaining her Orange Badge, and her taxi card.

'The others hardly see you once a month.'

'What could they do?` The whine again! 'They are all too busy. They go to work. You've got nothing else to do, and Victor lives too far away.'

'I saw you every week even when I lived in Purley,' I say. This was when I left that short second marriage, and ran to the house of my daughter Hayley and her husband.

'Well you must have enjoyed it, or you wouldn't have done it.'

No, Mother, you wouldn't do it if you did not enjoy it. I remember a day out with her and the children at Hampton Court. I did not have Imogen then, and Rafe was only three. We walked into the gardens and I organised that Mother take Anna and Hayley on the tour of the palace. Rafe was too young to do that, so I told Mother we would be outside when they came out.

'Are you going to walk round the gardens?'

'No I am going back into Bushy Park. Rafe wants to go on the swings.'

'Oh! I wouldn't put myself out like that for anybody.'

I clear up my dinner. I don't enjoy my soya meal, but it is cheap. Other meals might be as cheap, like fish fingers, which I do have as well and do enjoy, but they would not be as healthy. It would be nice to afford better fish or white meat so I could be healthy a bit more cheerfully, I think to myself. But as I am into health more than cheer, it has to be the soya rather than the fried egg. I am into anything that will make life better, for others as well as for myself.

*

When I ran from the abusive marriage I was in shock. I was in no fit state to handle the divorce, and nobody helped me. I think now that I was not really explaining to those who do love me just what was going on. It must have all been coming out scrambled. And so after that I was more than shocked. I felt like I was crawling along on my hands and knees, gasping for breath. Then, one day a spiritual book came my way. Whatever this tells us about the workings of whatever power; it was given to me by my mother who had found it in a jumble sale. It was called 'How to be Healthy, Wealthy and Wise.'
Mother probably thought it dealt with practical matters, and I doubt she had read more than the title for she did not refer to its contents. It was nothing like anything she has told me about from going to her Spiritualist Church.

The book was about a kind of spiritual life I had never heard of, and as I showed it to friends, more books came my way. Others came from spiritual and self-development courses which I took both for intellectual relief and as part of my search for healing. The message from them all is that we create our world and we can have anything we want if we truly believe that we can. It does not pay homage to any god person but to the power of the universe, a power that is in all of us. These books and courses have led me to practice

Transcendental Meditation, whose promise is that it will raise your consciousness to a higher level.

After my dinner and a few telephone calls to friends and children, I begin my meditation routine. The Ayur Vedic World advocates more than just the meditation. They claim that to progress more quickly, you should to do the full routine which begins with heating oil, then massaging that all over yourself, before doing some Yoga, then taking a bath, meditating last of all.

As I begin my yoga exercise, I wonder if my mother destroyed my sense of worth knowing that a poor self image would never attract a good relationship. Did she do that because she missed out on real sex as she missed out on travel, and just about everything else? As I stand in front of my full length mirror I think, no, not at all bad for my age, but I am not a teenager, and everyone says that is what every man wants. I think my body looks quite good.

Are my mother and I the same? Are we flowers born to blush unseen? I have had sex – I have children – but never satisfyingly, and now there has been 'nothing,' as my mother would put it for seven years. Not that I would count what was happening seven and a half years ago as 'anything.' When he touched me, I was screaming inside, because of the abusive way in which he spoke about women.
As I begin the process of oiling, I ache to have somebody touch me. I think of my mother enjoying 'been gone all over' by the nurses. The need for touch to me is sexual, but also part of a greater need for intimacy with another person, which above all means an intimacy of heart to heart. Maybe such is rare, between friends, relatives, and even lovers, and maybe it is that absence that makes us all increasingly as the philosopher says in his famous words: '... live lives of quiet desperation.' (Henry David Thoreau 1817-1862)

Then in the bath, I have to face that sexual un-fulfilment as a cause of my mother's generally disturbed state, is indeed only my interpretation, and that, in so assuming, I am projecting my own lack onto her. Maybe all she ever wanted was to travel, or maybe all she has ever wanted was to destroy somebody, for whatever reason, and found a possible victim in her first baby girl.

It has come to me how she must have looked on my face, even when just born (for she has told me that straightway I had a lovely face, and that the nurses took me round to show everyone on the ward). My face is still very gentle, and as a child it was very sweet – the little round faced toddler diligently bringing the tea without spilling – and she surely thought that here was somebody soft enough to manipulate, yet strong enough for her to lean on. Suddenly I remember what my son said to me on one of the many occasions that I said I wished I could make his Nanny happy. 'The only thing that makes her happy,' he said, 'is making you unhappy.' Well it certainly seems that way at times.

I wrap myself in cuddling towels and settle down to my meditation, hoping it will heal a lifetime of stress, and raise my consciousness to create only perfection and bliss. If only I could get Mother to do the same, but we are told by the Ayur Vedic world, that one person who is practicing Transcendental Meditation will affect, for the better, anyone close in their life, because their consciousness is linked.

Beautiful Dreamer

Chapter 13

It is Christmas Day and for the first time in years I do not have the digs about not coming to me for the festivities. None of us would risk Mother for any length of time now. She is so weak, and since the early near fatal heart failure which put her into the Home, we are all afraid. We have all separately taken her out for a few hours since she has been there, but the incontinence of many years is much worse. She has had accidents out with us, sometimes not just urinary, even with the Carers on hand to get her freshly padded up before an outing.

Still, a visit to Fawsett House does seem obligatory somehow, although in the last few years I have been free of Mother on Christmas Day. There are too many choices for me on that morning. The Unitarian Church I attend usually holds a Christmas Day service and that is at eleven in the morning, and I have a friend, who is alone at Christmas, and I do like to see her for an hour in the morning, but she is not an early riser.

What I often crave is to go to the open air pool in Hampton, which is heated, and open every day of the year. On Christmas Day, they serve a breakfast of salmon and champagne which is eaten sitting outside overlooking Bushy Park. This year I did ask my son to join me there as I do not want to go alone, but he says he can't. He is a school teacher in Hampton and says some of his pupils may be there. Anna and Imogen are teachers too, and they also avoid meeting pupils in the non-school world, such as in shops and cinemas.

I am always with my children on Christmas Day, one or all of them depending on whether any of them are going to their in-laws. We celebrate in all of our houses in turn, though it is usually in the house of Hayley and her husband, as that is the only place really large enough to hold us all. My three daughters are married and the older two have children of their own.

Yesterday I went to the Christmas Eve service at church, so today I visit my friend at ten thirty in the morning, arriving at Fawsett House an hour later. We do not have to be in Purley until one' o'clock. Hayley's husband is an actuary, as she was before she had a child. As I drive from my friend's house, only half a mile away from the Home, I remember how my mother used to irritate me by saying that her friend had a daughter who was an accountant just like mine. I felt as though I was banging my head against a brick wall explaining how being an actuary is much brainier than been an accountant, and more unusual. But I was wearing myself out, and thinking she is needling me on purpose, when she probably simply did not understand.

There is a big tree in the hallway of the Home, decorations are everywhere, and I can see long tables dressed with crackers in the conservatory where I normally sit with Mother. Gordon is already here, and soon Rafe joins us. My brother and all my children will be with me today. Although I live alone, I had a stocking to open this morning and have every year since I came to the house. My children fill it between them, hide it in my house a few days before Christmas, at a time they know I will be out, then ring me early on Christmas Day and tell me where it is hidden.

The Manager offers all the relatives a free glass of sherry. The staff at Fawsett House work throughout the year on a rota basis, which means they all in turn work on Christmas Day. One of the Carers tells me that the Manager is not officially on duty today, but that he always comes in for a few hours on Christmas morning.

Mother has many greetings cards and all her children have sent presents. I know that all my children have as well. Hayley is very generous to her grandmother, paying regular money into her bank account and telephoning her every week. Rafe presents Mother with a tiny radio. She already has one, but not that small, and she does like to take a radio right into bed with her at night, going to sleep with it, waking up to it. The new radio for the bed reminds me that she also sucks sweets in the middle of the night, and I think, not for the first time, how sad are her bedfellows.

One of the rare moments of mirth afforded by my mother, was to do with the eternal radio on in or by her bed. Soon after our dad died, she told us that ,one Sunday morning, she woke to hear hymn singing – and ` wondered where I was for the minute`!

We sit next to a resident who has a couple with her, who I assume are her children, or her daughter and son-in-law. 'How long has your mother been here? I ask.

'Oh, she is not related to us,' answers the man of the couple. 'My mother died here and we had got to know Ivy while we were visiting her. So we carried on coming. Ivy has no one else to visit her.' The couple joke about coming here, first for this one then for that one, until each one died, and that they would probably keep coming until they become residents themselves, perhaps not even notice the join.

Mother digs about me going off to my 'party,' with what I see as a cruel glint in her eye, as she pushes the guilt button in me yet again. Mother always came to me for Christmas Day in the early years when my children were young, but it was not a happy time as there was always some attack on one child being spoilt with what they had for Christmas, or one child being spoilt in the way they behaved. And, just as the children were playing with their new things, and we were settling down to watch something on television that we had looked forward to after all the cooking and washing up, then it would be, 'can't we go for a run in the car?'

I wish my mother well and so want her to be happy, but why have I never been able to explain to her what she does, and how she winds us all up? One Boxing Day I left my beloved Gilbert and Sullivan, which was on television, because she was fidgeting so much. Instead, I took her upstairs with me to bath baby Imogen. Another time, I remember the teenage Hayley arriving home after a day out with Mother, to please her, to please me, and being completely exhausted by the whole experience.

Of course I would like my mother with me on Christmas Day. I would like a cheerful, interested, and loving mother and grandmother to be in the midst of us and at our head. But as I pop into the visitor's loo by the entrance, before dropping my car home so that Gordon can drive Rafe and me to Purley, another Christmas memory comes to me. It was one Christmas Day when I was a single parent and Gordon brought Mother to us. All of a sudden at about 3'o'clock in the afternoon, he said that he had other people to call on. He would have to leave, and since Mother had no other way of getting home, she had to go too and, in effect, her Christmas was cut short. It was then that I decided I would learn to drive. Never would I be dependent on people ferrying me about at Christmas. And so, in spite of all the memories of my mother's visits to us and the horrors sometimes she made us suffer at Christmas, I have to remind myself that she has had horrors of her own.

Beautiful Dreamer

Chapter 14

'Do you want to borrow a comb?' This is Mother's welcome greeting on my first visit of the New Year. Funny the way she always goes on about my hair. She always had bundly hair in my memory. True, now, it is in the uniform 'set' of her generation, but in my childhood it was all done with rolls of hair in the front, secured by those small hair combs people wore, and quite messy.

I wonder why my hair has to be perfect, I think, remembering how Mother only had hers washed and set when she went to a hairdresser, and if she did not get there for a while, it remained unwashed. As she got older and life I suppose, more tiring, this happened quite a lot. Once I suggested she wash it herself, and she told me that she had 'washed the front'. Yet another moment of merriment provided by Mother as I pictured her walking about backwards, like a ham actor, making sure her front view only was on display.

Jogging myself back to the present, I realise that she has been at Fawsett House for seven months now, and she still believes she has only just arrived, and still wants to pack her things and leave. She demands her suitcases and begs for her shoes, yet again. How can I take her out with me in my car if she is wearing only slippers? A New Year, but nothing changed.

'We can't get her to take part in the Home's activities.' The Activities Officer comes to me and tells me how Mother will do neither flower arranging nor cooking. In fact nothing that is laid on to stimulate the residents.

'I don't want to be entertained,' she retorts. I try to talk to her about it, but the silence and disinterest hits me again. Over the Christmas period, I went to a party where I met a woman who sings, and presents concerts in Homes just like this one, so I have set the wheels in motion for her to visit Fawsett House.

It is obvious that Mother is becoming increasingly difficult, and I think that her 'entertainment' is being a nuisance to everybody, and maybe that has always been the case. The Carers tell me that she is bothering the other residents too. Usually, when I see her these days, she is almost alone in the large conservatory.

Most of the others sit in one of the smaller sitting rooms, one of which has a television.

Apparently, when Mother does go into these rooms, she gets hold of anyone who has an empty chair next to them, and proceeds to badger them with the fact that she is being kept here against her will and wants to go home, and, don't they think it is cruel that she is being imprisoned like this?

While still living in the community, Mother was seen on more than one occasion by a clinical psychologist, until she refused to go any more. I went to the woman myself for a while, giving details of my mother's life and lifelong problems, but without Mother's co-operation, there was little anyone could do for her, and anyway the psychologist told me what everybody else was telling me, there is nothing you can do to change someone of so great an age.

I could not accept this because of the spiritual teachings I was following. I could see no point in life continuing if there is no chance of inner growth. I even thought, in my mother's latter years, that maybe the reason why some people live so long when there is little quality of life, is precisely so that they can do the inner work that they have been avoiding for decades.

Hearing today how disruptive my mother is becoming in the Home, I wonder again why her Spiritualist Church did nothing, over the forty years she went there, to persuade her to make that inner journey. Once, I organised some relationship therapy for us both. As with the clinical psychologist, I went alone. Mother refused to go, and whenever asked why she would not go for counselling, said she had enough traumas in her life. I wanted to say to her that coming with me now might heal her trauma, but I was tongue-tied as always.

I sit with my mother having been told that she is becoming a troublesome member of Fawsett House, but know there is no point is discussing it with her. She cancelled the most recent psychology session because, as she said, 'I do not want someone coming and telling me I'm a terrible person,' and I wondered who had ever told her she was that. My father called me that, once. Perhaps it was him?

Then I remembered a time in my childhood when she had been on different occasions to a doctor about problems my brothers had, and that she had been told that it was all her fault. I am not going to ask why and how it is always the woman who is blamed and made the scapegoat. I am just angry. I was driven out of my house by abuse, but the man and some `friends` seem to put the blame on me.

I leave her amidst the usual complaints about not staying longer, not taking her with me, not getting her home. I am weary and in a hurry to catch the literature class that I attend, but the Activities Officer grabs me before I can press the code to get me out.

'I am using your mother as a case study,' she is saying to me, and I am thinking, aren't we all? She wants as many details of my mother's life as I can supply, right from her birth, as well as any clues about her likes and dislikes, her interests – anything which might help them find something to spark some enthusiasm in her. I make an appointment for a half hour interview next week and escape to my car, feeling released, but guilty about what I am leaving behind.

I am worried too that when I visit next week the visit will cut badly into my reading time for my literature class. Most of my adult life I have felt like this, that there are always callings on my time which prevent me from having a life of my own, or even becoming myself.

For one thing, it would have been relatively easy to have gone back to work after having children if I had ever had a proper job before, but to actually make a life from nothing takes enormous energy, and you probably need a long period of time to yourself in order to find a life, which is impossible when you are not only always busy but on top of that you are heaped with extras and emergences. And are always coping with abusive behaviours – from men, from relatives, from neighbours, and from so-called friends! Abuse drains the energy. Well, anyway, I have always felt as though I were drowning.

*

Another two months go by, and it is time for another three monthly review meeting with the officials at
Fawsett House.

These meetings are held in one of the smaller lounges of the Home, and as I enter I see that a circle of easy chairs has been arranged. Those present are the Manager of the Home, the Placements Officer for the Borough, the Social Worker from Mother's pre-Home days, Mother's Key Worker who supervises Mother's care, Gordon and myself. The clients themselves can attend the meetings if they so wish and we have tried with Mother, but at the first meeting she became very disturbed because as she said, 'everyone is talking about me.'

The Manager starts the meeting by summing up the past three months, stressing that Mother's harassment towards some of the other residents is becoming increasingly aggressive and disruptive. He has had several complaints about her. One client went to stay with her son and daughter in- law for a weekend and then refused to return unless my mother was removed.

'We simply cannot keep her,' he is saying. 'The other clients are verbally abusing her.'

'Not physically? asks Gordon.

'No, he replies, hesitating, 'but that could possibly follow.'

'She has a Personality Disorder,' he continues. 'In all my twenty years in this job, I have never met anyone like her.
What she really needs is one-to-one care,' he says, 'constant attention.` The matter has been discussed, but sadly the funding is not available. ` It is too late in the day to get her needs addressed now,' he continues.

'She needs to be in a place that can cater more than Fawsett House does for the mentally challenged.' The Placements Officer is talking now, and is saying that it could be some time before a bed becomes available in a suitable Home.

'Meanwhile,' says the Manager, 'we'll try our best to get her into the nearest of these Homes as a day visitor. That way she can get used to going somewhere else and we can see how she fits in.'

'She hears what she wants to hear, see what she wants to see,' explains my mother's Key Worker. 'She does not appear to listen, yet pounces on something you say, if it is what she needs to hear.' Of course, I have known this for years, and to hear someone else say it makes such a difference.

Mother creates her world out of limited ingredients, and refuses to allow anything else into the pot. I have suffered for many years, with her homing in on one small detail of somebody's behaviour to prove, for example, that my boyfriend was lazy or mean, or that my child is spoilt. We all live in our own reality world, but I have never been able to get anyone to see that in her it is extreme. Years ago when my mother was only sixty, I went to a counsellor and explained how talking to my mother left me feeling as if I was going mad.

'It is as though what she replies to me has nothing to do with what I have just said.' I explained. Now, at this meeting, the Placements Officer looks across the room at me, right into my eyes, and says, 'we want you to know that we know what is has been like for you.'

Just for that moment, it is as if a great stone has been lifted off my back. Here is someone, at last, whose knowledge of my mother is meeting me in what has been a very lonely place.

I drive home from the review, aware of a relief which has begun to makes its home in me ever since the nurse set me on a trail of understanding my mother. Now I have people who have experienced what I have lived with, and her condition has been given a name, 'a Personality Disorder.' I no longer have the self doubt I experienced when friends said, 'oh, well, your mum's getting on a bit now,' as if her behaviour was just to do with age and its attendant 'senility,' and not something that has been with her forever. The kind of place that my mother is to move into will be better trained to help, and now I have my own line of enquiry as I continue to talk to her. There may be some end, some peace, in sight.

'A Home more qualified in dealing with dementia,' the Manager said. So is my mother demented? This is not the usual old age dementia, senility, or Alzheimer's, for he said she has had a lifelong Personality Disorder, but does that mean, in a way, she has been 'demented' all her life?

I did spend a short time with Mother after the meeting, and the revelations of the meeting made me want to try yet again, to get close to her, or to what ails her, but as always I was greeted with the usual demands about going home to her mum. Still, that did give me a way in.

'But you didn't like it at home,' I said. 'You didn't like being with a mum who had to go in the shop.'

'I just wished I had an ordinary mum, that's all. One who could meet me from school.'

'You didn't like school much did you? I continued.

'I was too nervous. I wasn't clever at school. I couldn't do sums.' Well, that is part of the old, old story, I think, but then I got something completely new.

'... Those nuns, they could be spiteful, you know. The doctor told Mum to take me away from the convent. He said I was too highly strung.'

'What made you so nervy?' I asked gently.

'I was just highly strung, that's all. I can't help it. We are a nervy family.' Her dad had died of 'nervous debility,' I remembered.

'But something must have made you nervy. How old were you, when the doctor took you away from that private school?'

There was no answer. So I continued. 'Are you sure you were never abused?'

'No,

'No. Nobody hurt me.'

Chapter 15

Why did the Manager tell me my mother has a Personality Disorder, and then say she must go to a Home where the staff will be qualified to deal with 'dementia? I am confused, but I suppose these are all blanket terms – Senility, Alzheimer's, Dementia – all grouped together.

I am in the middle of changing the sheets on my bed and my mind is turning over the events of the day. I have just put the phone down after talking to Hayley, who is now at home all day with her little boy. She is not working, but using her time to attend a diploma course in psychology at Birkbeck College, and has just told me that there is new knowledge about Alzheimer's.

It transpires that the disease cannot be truly diagnosed until after death. The presence of the disease can only be proved when he brain is cut open, and more often than not it is revealed that the person did not have it at all. What is assumed to be Alzheimer's is often in fact depression, for the symptoms are much the same.

So, are most of the old people in these Retirement Homes depressed? And if so, what are they depressed about? Can Mother's behaviour be interpreted as some aspect of depression?

'She sees what she wants to see,' said the Key Worker, and she also called it tunnel vision. It is strange to me that she who would want to go round the world in a camper van or gypsy caravan, should be enclosed in such a tiny, tiny world, where history is comprised of Henry VIII and music means Madame Butterfly.

If only I had the ability to make everything all right. I have turned somersaults to do just that, tied myself in knots trying to understand her, just as I am doing in my attempt to put the clean duvet cover on, I think. In fact this is enough to make anyone depressed, I laugh, then it hits me.

I have a double bed whereas my mother has had a single bed for decades. Now, is that a difference of interest, or of hope? I struggle with the duvet and wonder what could be the root of Mother's problem.

Mother has always twitched and blinked. With some of her family they have the tendency to blink all the time, and rapidly, intensely. I recall a conversation, about blinking, which I had with a psychology student in my undergraduate days. He told me that this used to be called St Vitus' Dance, and some people think it began during the great plague of London.

'What would you expect?' he said. 'Everyone was dropping dead around you, and it could be you at any time. Wouldn't we all be twitching with nerves – with terror?'

Trauma. Post traumatic symptoms. Can they have been passed down through the generations and for so many centuries too? My mother's older brother had a deformed hand. He had two fingers joined as one big finger. Now, my older brother has a watered down version in that his two fingers were joined at birth. They were separated, but one finger remained shorter and without a finger nail.

So, old age dementia could be many things. It could indeed be the death of brain cells, which is what most people think. It could also be an inherited disturbance, or maybe a memory of trauma, which has been passed in the memory cells, which the Ayur Vedic world tell me are in every part of the body.

Thinking of my spiritual teachings I bundle the bedding into the washing machine and wonder about past life trauma. Are the demented recalling the shocks of the last life they lived, or indeed of any lives they have ever lived? What about the residents at Fawsett House? I have wondered if a lifetime of un-fulfilment or just plain old fashioned unhappiness grows like a snowball, gathering and gathering, until it is so great that you need to escape it by making up stories.

Dementia, depression, traumas, shocks. I suddenly remember the bomb. Mother was a small child during the First World War and her aunties told me that once a bomb landed very near to the shop in the East End. They claimed that her twitching began then. Shock could have made her twitch, but why was it never treated? Could it have been treated in those days?

I wonder, and I also consider that the bomb may have led to the behaviour which has driven anyone who knows her to near insanity themselves. Thinking about the bomb landing near

Mother reminds me of her family history, and that I once read that we can all bear the scars of second and third generation pain. Her grandfather was an aristocrat who was cut off without a penny for marrying the wrong girl. Could the financial loss, never mind the rejection and isolation from the family, be enough to reach as far as my mother, then on through her to me?

The murder mystery I have at the moment is particularly good, and I always look forward to my read in bed. A career analyst once told me that the things I like, or am good at, like crossword puzzles, poetry and detective novels, are all the same: analysis and detection. At school I was as good at Maths as English literature (and wish I had followed that path). Can Maths be a form of detection too – analysis, unravelling?

And I am trying to be a detective, in trying to work out what is the matter with my mother.

The appearance of the `Detective` is relatively new, and detection was in its infancy in late Victorian times. In 1906, Freud likened psychoanalysis to detective work. He says both activities are concerned with uncovering `hidden psychic material`, and that, ` in the case of the criminal it is a secret which he knows and hides from you, whereas in the case of the hysteric it is a secret ... which is hidden even from himself.`

I reach for some paper and an envelope as I want to write to Imogen this evening. I re-label an old envelope and put sellotape beside it, for sealing when the letter is written. I use old envelopes and skimp on food. I have my hair done and drive a car, but the hair is always done on special offer rates and I count the miles I drive, which is how I can afford a hairdresser and afford the stamps for letters to Imogen.

Of course, I shall write the letter sitting on my bed.

Beautiful Dreamer

Chapter 16

'Have you come to take me home?' It is my last visit to Fawsett House and we are three months on from the Review Meeting. The Placements Officer has finally told us there is a room for Mother in a Home in New Malden.

My story about the hair has come back from two magazines, and now I am getting an idea together for this book about my mother. Mother does not know what is about to happen to her. She has been going to another Home in Kingston, as a day visitor, and has complained all along about it, telling me that she is not joining any more 'clubs.'

At least there is a bit of entertainment in the Home for me today. I found Mother in a small lounge next to the conservatory, as that is in use. Through the glass partition we can see what is going on. Some Carers are having a lesson on how to use the hoist. This is a metal structure used for winching clients who are immobile up from their chair to a wheelchair, and from wheelchair to toilet or bed. There are many straps, as on a baby harness, which have to be properly put in place for the person to be safely lifted. Obviously new Carers must learn how to use this, and it seems that they learn by practising on each other. One is strapped in and the lever is cranked too fast, and she shoots up into the air. We can see the staff giggling, and I am guessing that this is probably a bit of intended larking as the cranking looked very hard and I doubt if they would normally be strong enough to shoot someone up into the air. They must need light relief as times, surely, in this place.

I look at Mother, but she is not amused. That does not surprise me. I tried hard enough always to bring her out of her misery, trying to bring some fun to our Sunday outings, but I rarely told her anything which made her laugh. Once, when I told her something funny that had happened to a friend, she looked at me and said, 'oh, so you've seen her again, have you? You see a lot of her, don't you?'

It was the tunnel vision again. Not that this was something hilarious to share, but it had been told to me by my friend, which meant that I had been giving my attention elsewhere, and I doubt if she had listened to the rest of the story. Once, I asked her why

she did not like me having friends, and she said that she just felt the friends were more important to me.
'I don't see my friends more than I see you,' I bleated, but she did not appear to hear me. Once she said she sometimes wondered where I got all my friends from, and I felt like I'd been to the 'Pick and Mix' friends counter, and been too greedy.

We are interrupted by the continual walker. We have been alone in this little side room, as most of the residents are in the television or quiet lounges, or even the bar. I expect that the closing of the conservatory has caused a bit of a pile up in these other places today. While watching the pantomime there, I thought I heard the harsh voice, and now she enters our room. Where she normally walks alone, this time she is in a crowd. They settle in chairs on the opposite side of the room to us, and huddle together in a 'cliquey' sort of way.

I am trying my hardest to get my mother to laugh at the antics with the hoist, but the voice reaches me.

'I had an abortion, you see. I had an abortion when I was forty-two. It was my hubby; he said we didn't have enough room. We already had three, and a tiny house. It was my hubby…it was he who made me have the abortion. I had an abortion when I was forty-two…We would have had room. I know we would have had room.'

So that is why she walks, I think, as I decide it is time to say goodbye to Mother. The walker is running away from her husband, she is running to try and stop him 'making' her have the abortion. Or is she running from herself, for allowing him to have his way?

I press the code, get outside, and think of all the clues I am being given in my search to find what torments my mother so, what causes her 'dementia.' That poor grizzle-headed soul who walks up and down on festering legs, with thick socks and old trainers, she hardly stops walking, yet she is not just senile.

There is a reason behind all 'madness'. So far the 'perfect figure' has made me think of Mother as a sleeping beauty; and so many stories tell me of the need in women to be adored. There is Mother's reference to the spiteful nuns, and that even in those days, a doctor had labelled her as highly strung and deemed her state of nerviness to be so bad that he recommend her to change schools. Then, I have seen the torment caused by a trauma, like a forced abortion.

I suddenly realise I am leaving this place for the last time, and turn from the door to go and offer my goodbyes to the Manager and the Carers, and something that has been at the back of my mind since I first saw Mother today, suddenly hits me.

She was wearing a new brooch. I thought I recognised it, so I ask her Key Worker. 'Oh it belonged to Grace. She died last week. Her family wanted to give some of the resident's items of her jewellery.' Grace who has 'not dropped' hers, I recall.

'And they thought your mum looked so alone,' the Key Worker is saying. So yet again I fall into the guilt whirlpool. I should be with my mother more. I should stay with her for a whole one day, I should occasionally stay the night, sleep beside her. The misery of self doubt engulfs me yet again. Could I have brought in a Spiritual Healer? A masseur? Or perhaps some soothing music? I feel time is running out for me to bring my mother to some kind of peace, but time is running out for me too. I want to become a successful writer; I want to meet a lover… I have needs too, and unhealed hurts.

Beautiful Dreamer

Chapter 17

'You leave me alone. I want to go home, leave me alone.' It is my first visit to Churchfield House and I can hear my mother's voice echoing as I walk into the sitting room, though she is nowhere in sight.

'She's being taken to the toilet,' says the Manager who greeted me and is now escorting me to where my mother will be returned.

Mother arrived here this morning, and the Manager has invited me to have lunch with her as it is her first day. I came and looked over the place a week ago and was pleasantly surprised at how luxurious it is. Mother's room is much larger than the one she had before and is on the ground floor with French windows opening out onto her own little patio. She even has an en-suite bathroom.

In the last place her room was upstairs and tiny, and she had to use one of the communal bathrooms and separate lavatories. Her place in both of these Homes has been funded by the local council, as she has never had any capital and only has her pension boosted by Income Support. Since she first entered Residential Care, I have been dealing with her debts, brought about largely by the number of taxis rides she took in the last year at home, when she was unable to walk to the bus, and the numerous phone calls she made in her desperate loneliness.

'I want to go home.'

At first, I thought the voice that greeted me was aggressive, but as it continues I can hear that it is full of terror. Lunch is in half an hour and I certainly have to 'sing for my supper,' but then haven't I always? I remember the free dinners I had as a bonus for taking Mother out all those Sundays, for the day.
The Sickness Benefit and the Income Support I receive now that I am signed off sick, amount to less than her State Pension topped up with Income Support, and I did not see why I should not allow myself to take 'expenses.' after all, I was not getting a fee as lady's companion, was I?

Coffee is brought in as Mother approaches me on her walking frame. Her progress is slow, and she is looking me full n the face, with hatred. We drink the coffee in silence and a resident comes and fiddles with our biscuits.

'That one is not quite the thing.' Mother speaks to me for the first time, and as we drink I began to notice the difference in this place. In the last Home, the other residents largely spent their time sleeping, or just sitting with lolling heads. My mother's words have always rankled, in that the content of what she says often bears no relation to what I have just said, but out of the mouth of the biscuit fiddler come words that have no relation to each other, and do not even make up a sentence.

The easy chairs are widely spaced around the room. The building has many units each with a lounge and a small kitchen for the making of tea and coffee. In each unit, bedrooms lead off from an open plan lounge and kitchen, and the cooking is done in a central one which serves the whole Home. We have been having coffee at a small table but now we move to one of the small dining ones and our cutlery is brought in. Mother looks across at me.

'I'd like a blouse like that,' this is the second time she has spoken to me. I am wearing a soft lilac coloured T-shirt handed down to me by Anna. It has a collar and little buttons and makes the best of my bust and blue eyes. We often pass clothes around in the family. Even my son got the shirt off my back in the form of a grey sweatshirt once. Feeling my children's clothes around my shoulders is comforting, like being embraced, like having them with me all the time.

'Can you get me one like that?'

'I'll try, Mother.' As plates of chicken casserole are put before us, I think how Mother always does this. Whenever she shows an interest in clothes, it is always because she wants what I have. Since my clothes are often from a 'Nearly New' shop, it is impossible for me to go hunting for a replica for her.

I remember some of the clothes shopping trips with Mother. As well as coveting what I wear, she has always hankered after what 'they' are all wearing. It may be the latest style in coats or a particular cardigan that is all the rage. I think of one particular desired item which brought about a trip to Kingston. `Everyone` was wearing a long cable knit cardigan in those days, with big buttons, and a same material belt, which you could let hang from its loops or tie around your middle.

I made the effort to meet her one day when my children were at school, and we had lunch first in British Home Stores.

knew there were lots of cardigans there, but as soon as I began holding the different colours up to her in front of the mirror, she was fidgeting and looking uneasy. Once I got as far as trying to get her to take her coat off so we could try one on for size, but she was troubled, edgy, and shaking.

'Let's leave it. Leave for now.' She became more agitated. 'No, no. I want to leave it now. I don't feel like it today. Don't feel like it today.' I could see that she was distressed. Was it because she did not want to be seen to be getting something she wanted as with the birthday presents, or was it that she did not want me to think she was all right now? Or was it the control thing again, and she wanted to control me to go shopping with her, but then felt that I was controlling her by making her choose one of the jackets?

Shopping with her has always been exhausting. In the days when she was 'enjoying herself' and she knew that I was 'not happy,' I met her most weeks with my second baby in her pram and my first little girl sitting on it. We would walk round the fruit market in the Market Place in Kingston, and then around nearby Woolworths, buying things I could only get there. Afterwards, we had tea in British Home Stores, which was next to Woolworths in those days, and had a café that backed onto the river.

After that, I would leave the girls with her and they played by the river. (What was I thinking – Mum and small children by an unfenced stretch of water?) I would take the pram, with its shopping tray underneath, to a small supermarket to get my main grocery shop of the week. While we had tea, Mother and I would sit opposite each other, the girls between us on either side.

Then she would go on and on at me about how poor I was.

Maybe I was, but I did not want it rubbed in. Did not want her gloating. I guess I was gobbling up any snack she cared to give me, partly because I was always hungry for actual food in those days, but also because I was so obviously starving for anything to be given to me by my mother. What she said felt like a rubbing in, that I was not worthy of getting a man who could provide for his family, that I was in no way lovely enough – woman enough – to attract a good provider.

To have explained that we were very young and that my husband earned very little, being as he was at the beginning of his career, and that with two children and consequently a non-working wife, there was naturally not enough money, but that in fact he kept nothing back and I held the purse strings, so it was not that he was denying me anything – would have been a total waste of time. Mother would not have believed me No. Would not have heard me.

All the time we had been going round Woolworths and the market, she had nagged me that my husband should do all the heavy shopping. Then, in the café there was this vicious attack. I remember feeling myself sinking down further and further in my chair. Couldn't I afford to have my hair done? It was awful that we never got out in the evenings. Could I ever afford a new pair of shoes? Did I have any pocket money? I felt like a worm, a slug.

And now this same mother is envying my T-shirt!

In the previous Home, when I stayed for lunch with Mother, she paid and we were served in the conservatory. Only once did we eat where everybody else ate, which was in a dining room with rows of tables. Here, this large room has easy chairs at intervals around the walls, and low tables near them for coffee, and small dining tables are positioned in the middle of the room for meals and for games, such as Ludo or jig-saw puzzles.

Some of the residents here are being fed by Carers and some are refusing to eat. This I did not see in the Retirement Home, I presume because it catered for those in the pre-dementia stage. Some here are also very agitated, pressing Carers again and again with the questions I heard as I had coffee with Mother. When was their daughter coming? What time was it? As lunch is cleared, one of the ladies asks a Carer what she should do now. 'Just relax,' is what she gets, and I ponder that the only needs recognised should be sleep, medication, food, toileting – and relaxing.

What about stimulus? What about understanding, and what about help with deeper problems? Like the problem of being so forgetful that you do not remember your daughter's visit, and are therefore perhaps feeling abandoned. Some games are resumed. Others sit and sleep, or just sit, or harass the Carers with endless questions or demands to be taken to the toilet.

It is time for me to go, but I know there is no point in suggesting to my mother that she joins in the games. Would I want to play Ludo? There were activities like flower arranging and Reminiscence groups in the last Home, and I have already investigated the extensive programme of things to do here, including sessions of gentle exercise. My mother has never been a joiner, has never really mixed with other people. She went to the Spiritualist Church but talked only of the healers and what they had said to her about whether she would win the pools, get a holiday, or come to live with me, and that they gave her a nice cup of tea.

However much she did not make friends through them, she always did enjoy coach outings and loved the trips arranged by the last Residential Home, where they did sometimes take their residents to the seaside. This Home has only opened as Mother arrives, and so far they have no plans to take their clients out. However, I have nearly got it together to bring my singer here.

Two friends were made on the coach trips of her early widowhood days. One she eventually gave up because the woman was always half an hour late for a meeting. The other she stayed with until the friend died. That one she visited in her house and was glad of the meal and the magazines given to her there. But she was not allowed to speak. The woman would say, ` no, you don't talk`, and did all the talking herself!

If you are in a world of bullying and abuse, it works both ways. I have tried to tell people who bully me that they are laying themselves open to the same by somebody else. Mother orders our times together, but there the friends controlled it all. Pity they did not keep their friendships to the coach outings only.

Mother always found it peaceful to be driven along in a coach or car. The way she spoke of the restfulness and the peace and tranquillity has always made me think that being driven was some kind of respite for her soul. Dad driving her along, or having a cup of tea made for her, gave her a feeling of being cared for I think. However, although she was always taken on some outing by her children, she never made us feel like doing more because of the way our offerings were received.

Hayley once said she would take her grandmother out for the afternoon on her birthday. All that morning, Mother kept telephoning me, asking when was my daughter going to turn up.

'I told you it would be in the afternoon, Mother.'

'Why can't she come earlier?'
'Because she is busy,'

'What's she busy doing?'

Chapter 18

I do have a lot of friends, quite an 'allsorts' selection in fact. They come from the many worlds of my interests, Adult Education, and the meditation world, as well as from the Unitarian Church. This church has no fixed creed, so fits my thinking exactly, where I am at, as they say, spiritually, as it is simply a place where beliefs can be explored. Mostly, I go for their discussion evenings, based on spiritual searchings, and personal development. The actual services I do not like so much and have only attended those on the specials days in the Church's calendar, taking Mother particularly at Easter or on Mother's Day. She never showed any interest in anything that was said in those services, but she did like it when the woman Minister visited her in her flat, and liked it even more when she got included in Church outings.

One Easter as we sat in the pub after the church service, she raised the question about the Easter message. 'Have they decided whether all that is true?' I really did not know what to say, though later I wished I had said to her that it is up to everyone, including her, to make up their own minds about whether the New Testament story is true. Once she told me I was 'biased' because I did not want to go to her Spiritual Church. Quite simply, anyone who did not think or believe anything that Mother thought, or believed was 'biased.'

My friends come from the many different classes I have attended or taught, and some are customers from my own small business which I ran for a short time. This was my own Adult Education where I got speakers in to give talks on a variety of subjects, the talk being followed by a social and discussion time.

The discussions are probably what I loved the most as I believe it is of enormous importance that people meet and share thoughts and ideas, a coming together of similar minds and maybe sometimes a flash of changed thought, of new insight. I also believe that a social time, with refreshments, helps towards this end. I do hold the occasional selling party, like Tupperware, or the selling of clothes or jewellery. This way, I bring together a group of women who come from all the different areas of my life, and so, over the years, they have mostly all met.

Beautiful Dreamer

Today I am having a clothes party, and so into my house comes the demonstrator, Hilary, who has become a friend through doing these shows. She has set up her wares on rails in my living room, and we have tried on clothes and chosen some. Now, we all sit enjoying a shared lunch to which everyone has brought a dish. Linda is here from the literature class I attend, and Naomi who has been in my life since we attended as assertion class together some fifteen years ago. Then there is Trudi from the church, and Betty from a past exercise class.

Over the quiche, salad and wine, I bring them up to date with my mother, and my quest to understand what makes her so unhappy. I tell them of the theory about her being abused as a child, because of the muckiness.

'I don't know,' says Linda. 'Michael and I had this friend, well acquaintance more like, who worked with Michael and kind of latched on to us. Did not seem to have any friends, bit of a loner, suppose. I always thought he was a bit of a nasty personally. Anyway, he suddenly married, and I admit I was a bit surprised, but he did meet her through an agency. Anyway, it didn't last long and he used to come round complaining how she was going to bed in a track suit, a dirty track suit, with dinner spilled down it. Then she started leaving dirty underwear on the bedroom floor, I mean, shit stained underwear. In the end she was even leaving shit on the bathroom floor, said she had diarrhoea, couldn't help it, and had not noticed she had left a bit.....'

'Is that what you call, smoking someone out?' asks Trudi.

'Well, she didn't. He stuck it out like glue. She had to go in the end.'

'So was it just a way of trying to get rid of him?' I suggested.

'Well, it was hardly trying to keep him, was it?' Naomi contributes..

'Trying to avoid sex, if you ask me,' says Hilary. 'Not exactly an attempt to turn someone on is it, the mucky track suit?'

'Well, it turned out,' continues Linda. 'When it all came out and she sued for divorce, that he was abusive to her, and was sexually sick.'

'So it was some kind of punishment?' asks Trudi.' Going to bed in the track suit, I mean.'

'Some kind of shock reaction' I suggest. 'She must have been in shock, finding what she had actually married.'

Is that what it was about, muckiness, I wonder, as I clear the table and begin making up the orders for clothes. Well, Mother was hardly trying to smoke Dad out was she? She did not even carry it through when she did run away. Now the avoidance of sex by making yourself unattractive, that I could understand.

I join them round the table with the order forms, and fill in my own, because by having the party I get a good discount. I tell them about the cardigan girl in the book I read and Naomi, who is divorced, says she can remember behaving like the cardigan girl too. 'It was just that I was never attracted to my husband,' she says. 'I guess we married too young because we both wanted to get away from home. I was ashamed of my breasts because I was hardly letting my husband touch me. I hunched my shoulders and crossed my arms and slouched. I actually did not want any man looking at my figure because I felt guilty – about having a sexy body on false pretences, I suppose.'

So then I tell them about the dress which Mother wore day and night, under her nightdress and under her day clothes. They all agree that that could have been to do with a fear of sexual advances, that she either found sex distasteful or feared another pregnancy – or both. We finish with cups of tea and all but Hilary leave. We settle the business side of things, then at last I am alone with my thoughts.

Have I got any further in my understanding of my mother? It all started with being told that she still has a 'perfect figure.' She showed an aversion to sex in my childhood, yet she stroked herself all over and liked, even enjoyed, being examined medically. She made a point of telling us when her sexual relationship with our father ended. There is the muckiness of her appearance and her habits, which my daughter with a psychology degree says are all signs of the sexually abused child, but my mother has denied that.

Now I am hearing stories of women hiding their sex through avoidance or fear, of behaving filthily out of hatred for a man who had abused and shocked. Did my mother hate my father for getting her pregnant and landing her in a life she had hated as a child and had wanted to escape? Surely there must be some sort of self-hatred in revealing your shit to the world, or even to one person? Especially if that person is one you despise?

I remember Mother's faecal accidents in our houses and cars, and I remember saying to Gordon, 'is she shitting on us?' But why would she do that? It must take an enormously low self-image for someone to abase themselves in that way.

On the other hand, even that could be worth it if it were the only way to show just how desperately in pain you are. Don't people shit out of fear? If so, was it fear of dying, or the memory of something too awful to tell?

Chapter 19

Churchfield House has actually got Mother doing something, an activity. This is an achievement. She has drawn a picture. The drawing is almost exactly the same as the ones she used to draw when I was a child. It is of a lady, side view on, head and shoulders only and there are those high cheek bones that she so admired in films stars. I say almost because the drawing is so thin, so light. The pencilled outline is so pale it is as though Mother were hesitant, did not like to press too hard; didn't want to make her mark.

It is Imogen's birthday soon and I spend half an hour with Mother. Instead of having coffee, we make the drawing into a birthday card. The piece of paper is large and the drawing on one side, so it is simply a question of folding the paper over to make it into a card. When she writes her name, I notice the pen line is feathery too.

Mother's handwriting has always been illegible, and has become increasingly so over the years. Now it is faint as well. It is as though this person who has never been able to communicate clearly what her wants or problems are, is now letting any impression, which she now has the opportunity to make, fade away too. It suddenly hits me that her speaking voice has indeed become very quiet a lot of the time, especially when she asks a Carer for our tea, or to be taken to the toilet. A light pressure with the pen, a hesitant whisper, is all hope giving up the ghost, of ever being noticed or heard?

I think of her wasted talent as I tell her that I must go soon because I am running my Creative Writing class in the afternoon, but then the old assertiveness returns, at least with me.

'Can't you be a bit late? she asks.

'No, Mother' I say, zipping up my large bag with the thin paper 'card' safely placed between the sheets of a notebook to keep it flat. 'Thank you for the drawing,' I say as I leave.

As I drive away I cannot stop thinking of her wasted talent as an artist, and the way she is so out of touch with the world of education.

'How do you know what to do?' Mother has asked me on many occasions about my Adult Education teaching, and 'how do you know what to say?' As well as teaching writing, I have published my own short stories and she has always asked, 'how do you think it all up?' In the days when she read a lot, she often said she would like to write a book, but that it would mean staying indoors, so she could never do it. Once, when I was reading for a degree, she telephoned my house when I was revising and said that it was a pity I had to stay in on such a nice day.

Gordon has been a Maths teacher for years and for the last few has been Head of Department. Again she has many times asked me how he knows what to say and what to do when he is standing in front of a class.

We know she was put down by her brothers and maybe that destroyed any chance of confidence with her school work, then the ignorance gained momentum from there on.

We also know that she was given a private school education for a few years and that she 'always had the best.' I know too that she had piano lessons, but she told me several times that when she played, just once, for our father, soon after they were married, he laughed. And she never played the piano again.

My father had little education but was a talented man. He played the piano himself, by ear, so why did he need to put her down? Was it because he was not able to provide well for us? Was it a way of dealing with his own personal guilt at getting her pregnant and so trapping her in a life of poverty? By putting her down was he able to put her into the role of 'the stupid one,' so that he could say everything was her fault? Did doing that make him feel any better? Is that what she is doing to me, putting me down to make herself feel better? Can she focus on my stupidity and so forget the 'silly little Nellie' role dumped on her? A spiritual healer once told me that my mother is only doing to me what has always been done to her.

As I unpack my bag, glad that I cleaned and polished the house yesterday for the class will soon be arriving, I look at the drawing and wonder again at the light pencil touch which is hardly there. My mother, who has so much to express, yet is unable to get it out and show the world what she has to say, or what she has to give. If ever she was in my house when my children were studying for exams, she would say that they would 'wear their brains out.'

I wonder if that was some idea in the air, some idea given out by a suggestion in women's magazines, or on the radio? Did it come from the Church? Or was it just handed down traditionally from grandmothers and mothers? Was it some idea to keep women down? And men of a certain class too? To prevent them from becoming educated, to keep the status quo? For this is what I believe to be the root aim of our culture. And the cause of all ills.

Mother certainly grew in a small pot, but she had no chance of expanding because her bud was frozen from the start. Most of my activities are cerebral and are not dependent on travel. I can write and discuss anywhere and would rather have an exciting time in my head in a slum, than have nothing but boring conversations in a palace, or indeed while travelling the world.

Maybe this is partly due to my agoraphobia, which in me manifests as a fear of open spaces, which is how most people interpret the word. However for me it can also be anything from a fear of going out or being somewhere I have never been before, to making a difficult journey where I am not sure of the route. It can even take the form of refusing to go to specific places where I have felt indescribably and unexplainably ill.

Perhaps it is simply that I was too much 'out and about' as a child, with a mother who has always been claustrophobic and restless. Mother would not be able to sit still long enough to study or to write a story. She could not sit to feed a baby, and always said that she did not breast feed her children because she was too restless and `could not sit still long enough.` When she gave a baby its bottle, she put it in the baby's mouth, in the pram, the bottle propped up on a pillow.

I recall one Sunday arriving to take her out for the day, not from my house, but from my brother's house where I had been house and cat sitting for Gordon, while he went skiing.

'How often do you have to feed the cats? Mother asked as we set off.

'Twice a day,' I replied.

'You can always put out two lots in one go,' she suggested.

The cats wouldn't go near the food if a fly had been on it, and there was more chance of that happening if the food had been sitting in the corner of the kitchen for twenty-four hours rather than for twelve. I nearly asked her if she would like it if a Home Care assistant were to come in every morning and lay out five cups of tea, some toast, a plate of dinner and something for supper – all her food for the day going cold.

But was her life in some way just like that? In some way – metaphorically – was it nothing but cold toast and cold tea?

To some it might look like I have a good life, with classes and clothes sales and lots of friends. Yet, in a different way to my mother, all that is a running away even though it can take place in my own house. It is a running away from me, my true state, and avoiding the pain at least for a while.

When not engaged in activities, I swim alone, shop alone, clean the house alone, go to bed alone. When my mind is not busy with others I am in a black hell. I grieve for my many lacks and then grieve even more for the cause which is the failing of the law to look after my interests. Most of all I grieve my sex life, which has been so poor and now does not exist.

Then I hate my mother for all she did to make me the person who attracted such ills. Still I feel great sorrow for her. She has lacks too and I want to understand why she is as she is.

I can see the first car drawing up, my class is arriving. When it is over, I will do an hour of my own writing. Then I will retire to my bedroom to eat, telephone Imogen, do some yoga, bathe and then end the day with my Transcendental Meditation and pelvic floor exercises.

Chapter 20

'I want to go home.' I get the usual greeting as I walk up to Mother on my weekly visit. I have tried to get Mother to draw again, so that like me she might make her own greetings cards. My singer came to Churchfield, and I did manage to get Mother to see the show, although it meant I had to be there too. I also noticed that she joined in the singing, perhaps because there was no 'Daisy, Daisy.' But she resumed her fretfulness as soon as it was over, and the requests to go home are now becoming more insistent.

I still want, and hope, to make things better for her, and in so doing, bring about some measure of peace. I still dream of taking her to France – somehow – and sometimes talk to the people at Churchfield about the possibility of getting a masseur in, but I do not know of one, and neither do they.

The problem appears to be that there would be so much arranging to do in terms of co-ordinating my time, that of the masseur, and the space within the Home, as both the available rooms are used for other activities. Then, would an ordinary bed be suitable for a masseur to work on? What about her back? It seems that everything I want to do presents me with insurmountable problems, but how I would love her to be rubbed all over with soothing oils while healing music played in the background.

Imogen writes lovely, newsy letters to me, and puts a great deal of thought into them, but I feel that I do not give her enough of myself in return, even in letters or on the telephone. Life continues amidst all my various classes and 'Keep Fit' routines, and I occasionally send off a new story, and get it back. I am ploughing my way through the book, I have to remember to do my face and pelvic exercises. I long for the love of a man, but most of all I am exhausted. Gasping.

Mother is still harassing the Carers about letting her go home. They are extremely busy today, and we get no offers of tea or coffee. Usually there is a minimum of two Carers to each unit, and as I sit down with Mother one of the Carers takes a resident to the toilet. The remaining one comes up to me, and looks anxious. Another resident wants to go to the toilet too, and she asks me if I would keep an eye on all the others while she attends to the task. I give Mother the magazines I have brought for her and some chocolate, and while she flicks through what she has for years called 'books' she begins tearing at the wrapper on the chocolate. I look around at my charges, and wonder about their lives and how I could help.

There are several walkers here at Churchfield, some are what I call cardigan girls, shuffling along slowly with head and shoulders drooping and clasping the two edges of their woollies across their chests. The top of their bodies seem to me to be concave, with the heads and stomachs being the pointed ends of the half-moon shapes. One is walking ram rod straight. She is coming directly towards me and I feel threatened by what I feel is her menacing stare. She turns away only at the last minute before hitting our table, but she still treads stealthily, as though creeping up on somebody.
She is so straight down her face and her front, that I am reminded of the playing card soldiers in the Alice in Wonderland film.

'Mum wants me to go home,' Mother tells me quietly. 'I phoned her, but while I was on the phone I heard a voice telling my mother to keep me here.' So she believes there is a conspiracy against her now. I watch the 'playing card' lady and look at my mother and wonder what has demented them.

'Every time I ask if I can go home, they tell me to ask my daughter. They say it is up to you.' I try to interest Mother in a large print book that I found in a Charity Shop, but she pushes it away.

'Look, it is about history. A story set in the Middle Ages,' I tell her. She pushes it away and looks round the room. The two Carers are back, and Mother sees them and asks me if I would like a cup of tea. 'You must want a cup of tea,' she insists, until I say I don't mind. 'Will you make my daughter a cup of tea? She speaks in the direction of the Carer, but if anything the voice is much quieter than when she is talking to me, certainly a lot softer than when she is demanding suitcases or to go home.

'Can my daughter have a cup of tea?'

'My daughter wants a cup of tea.'

'Cuppa tea. Cuppa tea.' She asks, but not in a way that can be heard. I am surprised. It is that swing again, between rebellion and submission, between treating herself to café cakes and films, then abasing herself and bowing under the back bashing. She is asking but not asking for she does not say it in a way that can be heard.

Her voice reminds me of her drawing, which looked as though it were made by somebody nervous and afraid to make their mark. Look what happened when she did? The handwriting must have been sufficiently legible for her letter to be printed in a newspaper, but that brought her only derision and abuse. Was this the reason for the soft pencilled drawing? Is illegible writing some kind of block between herself and the outside world, like not joining clubs and making friends? A fear of what she might reveal of herself?

Is she almost saying, I won't present myself for scrutiny by mixing or speaking out, or write something that will be read?
Or is the message that she wants to communicate, but does not expect anyone to read or hear her, so she won't even try?
Is she trying to say that `nobody will want to hear what I might have to say,' or 'I can't possibly say what I need to say?` or perhaps `I don't know what it is myself`? I remember Freud and the ` secret hidden even from` ourselves.

Asking for the tea, is Mother acting the frightened little girl who asks for something, but does not want to be a nuisance – knows she must not trouble anybody, speaking it but hardly saying it?

I get up and have a word with a Carer and go into the kitchen which is off the sitting room, and make us both tea and biscuits. If only she would read, I think. If only she would take part in activities. It would keep her off the Carers' backs for at least some of the time. But of course, what I really want is for something to make her move, to improve, to reach some slightly higher spiritual state, to reach serenity and peace.

Over our drinks I tell her that the activities are not all cake making, there are other things too, like reminiscence where she could talk about her life, about the shop, about the past.
She has been persuaded to go to the activities room a couple of times, but has always left after a few minutes. Of course, one

look at the cake making session would have been enough to send her back to her lonely seat, and her lonely world.

As a result she would have seen the activity sessions as something out to get her, to force her into being domesticated, and to make her do things she does not like to do. I guess the domestic angle must have been what made her choose to avoid what was socially available to her when a young wife, which was the Woman's Institute. She told me once that was all 'embroidery and jam making.'

She hated the domesticity forced on her by motherhood, but her behaviour is also about control. She has viciously thrust away anything which she sees as control of her. Was that what the nuns did? Did she see them as 'spiteful' simply because they were in a position to make her do what she did not want to do? Always, Mother has believed that the kind of women who went to the Women's Institute would have been 'common scrubbing women' with 'nothing in their heads,' not like her. She had music and history in her head, she did.

'There are reminiscence groups,' I say again. For her to begin talking about her life must surely bring some kind of change which might set her on a growing path. 'You could all talk about your time in the war', I say. 'Lots of them here must have lived through the two wars, just like you.'

'I don't want to talk about the war,' she says, and I recall how, on the few attendances she made to a Day Centre in her pre-residential days, she was 'made' to sing wartime songs, like 'Daisy Daisy,' which she hated. She would far rather have sung a Beatles song any day, she told me. She did love the Beatles. Well, they appeared in the sixties when she knew I was not happy but she `was enjoying` herself with me dancing attendance. `Daisy Daisy` was the war, the Beatles represented what were perhaps the happiest days of her life.

'Don't they understand,' she says now, 'that most of us want to forget it?` I know Mother was terrified in the war. She said that the only thing she could think of was all the little children being bombed, and the longer it continued the more out of her mind with terror she became. Many times I have heard how she believes that she had a breakdown while expecting me. She could not stay in one place, and left my older brother with her mother.

Nobody expected me to be normal. Towards the end of the pregnancy, she was running all over the place, on buses and trains, as if she were trying to escape the bombing, not even combing her hair.(And now she nags me about my scruffy hair.) 'Is she all right?' was the first thing my dad asked when I was born.

They say that one trauma re-opens another. A death can bring back the experience, all the feelings, of a previous one, and a second divorce re-awakens the pain of the first. Mother had suffered the First World War and the bomb that fell nearby where she lived. She had a mum who kept going in the shop, and those spiteful nuns. She had been through a pregnancy when she was not married. And of course there is also whatever else that has not yet been uncovered.

'Some people enjoyed the war,' she has always insisted.
'Some women enjoyed having their husbands away. They went out with soldiers.'

'Why didn't you?' I asked.

'I didn't want to. All I wanted was all of you.' Well, she would not have wanted 'that nasty business,' would she? The business that she claims only brings drudgery. It seems she does not understand that some women have a sexual need, and even a driving desire for that to be satisfied.

I am back from the Home, and put the large print book by my front door, ready to return to the Charity Shop. I have my lonely evening ahead of me, of soya meal, yoga and meditation. But also – joy! I remember that I have a crossword. I picked up an old newspaper when I was last with Anna, and the crossword had not been filled in.

Mother has never understood why I have had men in my life, or is it that she resents them being there, taking her place? 'I can't understand why she has him to stay the night and not me,' she once said to my sister.

'Because he doesn't click his teeth, Mum, that's why,' was what Valerie told me she replied. But I don't think Mother would have heard, let alone understood. There was no answer to her question; to her I was just a failing daughter not having her to live with me.

'But he is in your house,' she attacked me once when one man lived with me for a while. I use the word attacked, but she also sounded baffled. 'I don't understand why you have him to live with you and not me.' Did she not really understand a woman's basic needs? Although she did not want sex herself, she must have seen plenty of evidence that a lot of women do. I remember one day when I was about ten, I heard my parents shouting at each other.

'At least she was a proper wife.'

'Well go back to her then.'

The next indication I had that my father was not happy in some kind of way with Mother, came about a year after that scene. It was a half term holiday and I went to meet him at the shop where he then worked. It was his half day, and we were going to see a performance of 'The Yeoman of the Guard,' the first Gilbert and Sullivan work I ever saw. It was my father who introduced his children to those operettas, and I will always be grateful to him for that. Mother did not like his music, calling Beethoven, Mozart, and Handel, 'his horrible dreary, music.'

This performance was going to be performed in a theatre on the pier at Southend. Having moved from the East End when I was nine, we had now lived near Southend for the past two years. Dad managed a shop there and we lived in a village a few miles away in a house bought by 'Jack,' Mother's mum.

When I arrived at the shop to go to the show, I found one of the shop ladies was coming with us too, and in the theatre Dad gave her a box of chocolates.

'Don't tell Mum,' said Dad. About the chocolates or the lady? I was more upset about the chocolates than the lady.

Through all our childhood we had a Dad who worked in a shop that sold sweets and chocolates, and part of that time we lived over the shop, but we never received a free sweet. My mother certainly never did, and some years we didn't even receive an Easter Egg, not even a small one.

It was much later when Mother told me that for many years Dad had been going out on his own on New Year's Eve. We never celebrated the occasion together as a family, and I guess I must have been in bed and not noticed his absence. I may have even thought that he was in bed before me, because he normally went to sleep very early because of the early start with the newspapers.

As I clear my dinner and get ready to begin the oil and yoga part of the Transcendental Meditation routine, I wonder if Mother had been hinting that Dad was out with a woman on those New Year's Eves. Since he told my mother she was not a proper wife, and took another woman out to that show, I guess it is highly likely that this is what was going on.

Yet I am still convinced my mother did have some sexual longing, albeit subconsciously. What about the touching herself all over? What about her announcing to her daughters that sex was over in the marriage? Then I remember a conversation I had with her in her seventies – years after her telling me that she had not wanted to go out with soldiers like other women whose husbands were away in the war.

It was when she had been having a moan about there never being any seats left for her on the buses, and how she hated the `hard faced old women` who had got there first and had taken them all. 'And I tell you what,' she said, 'I bet those hard faced old girls are the very ones who went out with the soldiers.'

But I thought you didn't want to? I reminded her.

'No... but it would have been something to remember, wouldn't it? She said wistfully.

Still I do not feel that I have got to the end of my search to understand her sexuality. Is she the Sleeping Beauty suggested to me by the nurse's words, and is she demented now because of her lost chances? Has she been a nagging shrew, or worse, did she have a severe Personality Disorder, because there was always that lack in her life?

Did she treat me in a way that destroyed my confidence so that I would never become a fulfilled woman, because she was not? Was she not interested in sex because she was with no 'Prince Charming' whose kiss could awakened that something special in her – and who also did not provide the crystal coach in the form of a gypsy caravan or a camper van?

Maybe it was simply that sex brought babies and drudgery, and she rejected my father because all sex meant for her was the rough end of womanhood, the labour pains and the endless nappies, with none of the glamour which makes a woman feel she is cherished and valued?

She had her first baby only days after getting married, and that to a man whose divorce had only just come through in time to honour her state. She spent the end of her pregnancy in an Unmarried Mothers' Home, which we now know to be places of punishment and degradation. She often told me that the birth was long and that no kindness was shown to her.
However, she also complained that throughout that long labour she was not even offered a cup of tea, which made me wonder whether it were particularly painful after all. Tea is not much on most women's mind when giving birth.

Nevertheless, she said it was bad, and birth usually is fairly so. Fathers were not present in those days, yet if she ever expressed any dread of an approaching confinement, my father would tell her that having a baby was only like shelling peas. When she told me this, I thought, yes, if you are prepared to throw away the pod! How did he know what it was like for humans? And anyway, society needs its husks, doesn't it?

When she found herself pregnant for the fourth time, she really did not want to go through with it. She was in her late thirties by then and told me that she was always very tired.
Nobody recognised how tired she was. They were all too busy criticising her for not looking after her children as she should. But a few years later she was diagnosed with severe anaemia and the doctor said he had only just caught it in time.

No wonder she went to a doctor in despair over this pregnancy and he prescribed a pill to end it. No one will ever know how weary she possibly was. I don't know how many times she said to me when I was a child that, in Sweden, if a mother gets too tired, she is sent away for a rest. She took the pill the doctor gave her and that night she lost the foetus, which was large enough to be seen, and be recognisable as a baby.

'Did you see it?' I asked when she told me. 'Did it upset you?'

'No, but Dad saw it. It seemed to upset him a bit.' Again I get a vision of some sweetness, at least, a shared sadness, between them. She went into hospital, and that was when my father told me that if Mum died, it would be my fault.
However, losing the baby upset her enough for her to want another, and so Gordon was born a year later.

A wanted baby that we were too poor to afford and there was a couple who lived across the road from us who had one daughter but could not have any more children. They asked my parents if they could adopt the new baby. My parents seriously considered this. 'We love you,' my Dad said, holding my tiny baby brother. 'But we can't afford you, so we are going to give you to Aunty Phyllis over the road.'

Why was I always alone in the kitchen when things happened? I witnessed my father bashing my mother's back.

I heard him tell my new baby brother we could not afford to keep him and would have to give him away. Frozen, I stood there listening, and the words tore at my eight year heart. I adored my little brother.

Beautiful Dreamer

Chapter 21

My father was clearly a talented and able man, yet he had a poorly paid job, had no success he could claim, and had to dump his self-esteem somewhere. He passed it on to my mother by blaming her bad management for the way we lived. He pushed his guilt about that pregnancy onto my head, and once when I said I wanted a new dress, he told me that I did not deserve it because I was a 'terrible person.'

Dad was an orphan and uneducated. He made pregnant a girl whose family owned a business and which also had claims to come from the upper classes. No wonder he let himself be bullied into managing a news agency when what he really wanted to do after the war was train as a chiropodist. Then, he produced a family too big to support on his wages, and must have felt a failure, especially with a wife who constantly nagged for a better life.

Surely it is not totally unrealistic to say that he could have produced fewer children? Instead of being aggressive when we asked for anything, he could have admitted to us that he could not afford the things we wanted and explained that this was the way of the world – where some jobs bring in less money than others, so some people have and some have not.

Perhaps in a different marriage he could have worked on the budgeting with his wife, even enabling her to find some way of earning money herself. As it was, when she once said to him that she would have to do something to bring in some money, he said, 'what could you do?' It was as though he was laughing at her, like he did with the piano playing. He crushed her as he felt crushed himself.

I feel now for his inner pain, for the loneliness of his life.
He did not have a loving marriage, or a happy sexual one. He worked long hours for little joy. His children thought him a mean man who was usually grumpy and sometimes frighteningly angry. I always thought of him as having big, scary, bulgy eyes. No wonder he took refuge in his beloved Beethoven, Mozart and Gilbert and Sullivan. No wonder my mother stayed downstairs on her own, doing the pools and writing to the Queen, hoping and dreaming of a better life.

My dad was funny too at times, and might have been different had his lot not been so rotten. Oh, given we had been together in a later age. I do wish now I had been able to talk to my father. He was horrible to me all the time I was trying to get to University. A few times, when he saw me doing my homework, he said to me, `I might not let you go.` and I believed he had that power.

That is unforgiveable. I had nowhere really satisfactory to do my homework. I was exhausted, and wanted so much the chance of a better life – and to take my mother round the world. Then to have hanging over me the threat that it could all be taken from me at the last minute. I think if asked to describe my overall life in one word, it would be ` exhausted.` Gasping for breath.

But when we were younger, he used to tell us a story. It was about the time when he got up early for work before the family awoke. He told of a little mouse who came to talk to him every morning, wearing a tartan waistcoat and a straw boater and carrying a cane. That is all I remember of the mouse, but oh what a dad was locked up behind his defences caused by his own low esteem and misery.

He tore off the top of one of my school reports, where he English Language section was, and the best report I have ever had. It must have been on the mantle-piece near the spills, and he used it to light his pipe. He also `mislaid` a letter which informed my mother that she had won a competition. (She had won it by making up a slogan. She was a one for words and I believe that she gave me my affinity for language.)

Two parents with untapped talents, who could have done so much more for themselves. For each other, and for us. Why don't people?

*

'I'm not going,' Mother greets me on this visit to Churchfield House. I feel angry because I have come especially, made a special effort, having told her last week that I would spend extra time with her by joining in the reminiscence part of the Home's activities. She said she would go, and the Carer's have been talking to her about it all morning and reminding her that her daughter is coming to help with the session. Now she is not going. She is adamant, closing her mouth in a determined line.

I have a cup of coffee with her and continue with the persuasion well into the time when the session would have started, then as I gather up my things to leave, I realise I was quite looking forward to the session too. It would have been like being back running a proper Adult Education class again.

Driving away, I am thinking that maybe there is something threatening about the suggestion of a reminiscence group, akin to the way some people fear any kind of counselling. I think it is the fear of being revealed, as if a long hidden goblin is going to make his appearance, like a monster from the past, and silently ever present, but whom they have never faced.

*

'I'm not going. I am not going.' Those words bring back memories as I arrive home and deal with answering machine messages and the post. The Unitarian Church I go to has at last found a Minister, having been without one for six months.

The Church Newsletter also tells me that there is to be a new venture after the service every Sunday, Circle Dancing.

They used to hold these dances a few years ago, when the past Minister was there. I remember trying it as a way of filling a Sunday, taking mother who enjoyed sitting and watching. It was a change from the usual round of coffee, lunch, shop and tea routine. I did not enjoy the dancing much, the steps were difficult and I found the whole thing boring. Maybe that was because my main purpose in going there was in the hope of meeting a man.

Her behaviour today has reminded me of another Sunday morning. It was summer and we had not had a trip to Worthing for some time, so that the nagging had been getting louder and more insistent. This was in the days of my last divorce, which went on for over a year, when my work was fizzling out and I felt I should make the week as much like a working one as possible.

I tried to make my mother see that the week had to be like a working one for me, more structured. As well as applying for jobs and sometimes going for interviews, I did not want to get out of the working day routine. The application forms, plus the endless other forms I seemed to be having to fill in for Mother, were more than enough to do, with my swimming and the one private class that had survived.

So, in spite of the complaints, I had held firm that if she wanted to go to Worthing it would have be at the weekend, albeit it was a struggle with the insistence that the coach would be too crowded, Worthing would be too crowded, she wanted her usual Sunday outing with me and felt that Worthing should be an extra. Surely I could give my mother an extra day, just for once?

I got up early that morning as I was living some distance from her, in fact at that time I was living under the same roof with my ex-husband in Teddington. Due to the recession, the house had not sold and the law had insisted that I should go back or I might end up losing my share of the property. In spite of the fact that I had spent nine months in Purley with my daughter, the man was not made to get out, in what might have been seen as 'his turn,' and so I was living with him and trying to cope with the abusive behaviour I had run from. I was in no state to stand up to Mother as well, so that Sunday I had got up at six to get ready and deal with a few other things, since I was losing a whole day.

At eight I was ready to drive to her. I needed an hour to pick her up, drive to Surbiton, drop her at the pickup point, and go off to park somewhere, walk back, and then probably be forced to have a cup of coffee in the café next to where the coach would come in. When I phoned at eight to say I was leaving, I was greeted with, `I am not going.' It would be too crowded, and anyway she wanted to go on Wednesday.

So I said, all right, and still took her out all day for the usual Sunday outing. Why did I do it? To have gone to her flat and dragged her to the coach would have brought more abuse.
She would have not have been clean and tidy and she would have refused point blank to get into the car.

I can see that nobody would understand why I then agreed to take her to the sea on Wednesday, since in a way she had missed her chance. Most people would have stood their ground and said the Sunday outing was instead of Worthing.
However, I knew full well the kind of abuse I would get, and the number of telephone calls, so I gave in about Wednesday.
What I do not understand is my taking her out on that Sunday.

I could have said 'OK, you won't go today, so I'll see you on Wednesday,' and put the phone down.

I am trying so hard to understand how she was able to bully me. Yes, I allowed it, but she also created that in me. Years previously Victor had invited her to go to him and his wife and son in Farnham for Mother's Day. He would pick her up and that meant a much longer car ride than she would ever get with me. But she was 'not going.' She called me and announced it on the telephone.

'Why are you telling me?' I was baffled. Why was she not calling Victor? The complaint was that Victor should not have to have her. I should be taking her out for Mother's Day. I did stand my ground on that one. After all, I was a mother too, and had been invited to lunch by Anna and her family. But the way she punished me for that outing with Victor made me think of a child grizzling because its mummy has sent it to be looked after by Aunty. Basically, the message was that I was `fobbing off' my duty, as when she said I would want her to remarry so that I would not have to look after her.

How many times has my mother almost, emotionally at least, stamped her foot with an 'I'm not going`? When that last divorce was over and I no longer lived in Teddington, I stayed briefly, between houses, with my younger brother who lives in Epsom. Some of my mothers' family, especially Gordon and my daughter Hayley, have always worried a lot that my mother has not travelled, as she always wanted to.

Now, because I was living with Gordon, I was able to talk about our mother at length, and said how good it had been of him to take her to France just a day once to Calais, and how it grieved me that she had not, as she always put it, 'seen the world.'

Gordon said he was prepared to take her on another day trip, perhaps to Boulogne but that, now that she was older, and frail, he would need me to go along as well, in order to help him with her. He knew my financial state and said that he would not expect me to pay. When I told mother of the proposed outing she was excited, but when she heard that I was going too, she must have guessed Gordon would be paying for me, knowing I had no money.

`Then, I'm not going,' she said.

She was prepared to deny herself this treat because I must not be treated too. How I saw it was that she was controlling the status quo: I must not move out of the role of the person who does not have things, even if that meant she lost her chance to go to France.

Strange that to keep me where, for some reason, I had to be should make her feel better. Strange that she was prepared to forgo a treat for that purpose. For thirty years a widow, she scarcely had a holiday. There was another one I organised for her – through some Charity or State aid – in this country it is true, on the coast and too far for me to drive.

Gordon was prepared to drive her one way, my sister and her husband the other. My sister likes to get out as our mother does, and for her it would have been the excuse for a weekend away. But, again, Mother was not going. Not if `everyone has to be routed out.` She would have gone if I had done the two trips.

It was during that stay with my brother, when the day to France was suggested, that the first of her brothers died, and Gordon said he would drive her and me to Essex for the funeral. I got countless calls about taking her shopping for a smart jacket. Finally at the end of a divorce and homeless period, I was in that stage of house buying which is often fraught, with problems appearing as a result of the survey, and speedy negotiations required. The calls from Mother came like persecution. In the end, she came to the funeral in a hotchpotch of colours, and a cardigan instead of a jacket.

The message was clear. If I didn't dress her then she would show us all up. She always wanted me to dress her, giving time to her when my daughters got married, more than to them

I was always meant to be, as well as her daughter, he mother, her husband, her sister, her cosy aunt and her buddy friend – her Lady`s Maid.

Another time, instead of the 'I'm not going,' it was as though she had spat in the face. It was not literally a spit, but it felt like it, as did all those other refusals. In the early years of my first divorce, one Bank Holiday my eldest brother invited me with my children to visit him and his wife, and also invited Mother.

I had no car so Victor came to pick us up, having collected Mother the day before, to give her a longer weekend away. As soon as I walked in she looked away from me and turned her face pointedly in another direction as we walked through the door. Sideways, she said to me that Victor would have taken her out for a drive, but now there were too many for the car.

Another of the few remarks directed at me was to ask what the man in my life was doing that day, which I took as a comment that meant I was my boyfriend's responsibility and I should be taken out by him and not by my brother. I felt I would be wasting my breath trying to explain that I had come to see my brother, not just to have an outing.

Victor whispered to me that he would not have taken her out for a drive anyway. He was driving a lot in his job those days and got tired of driving. I wished he had said it to Mother, but she would not have accepted it if he had. It would have been an 'excuse' and the truth was that I had 'got round him' and persuaded him to invite me.

She also glared at Rafe, that day, when he was eating. He was putting on weight and ate a lot in those days – maybe as compensation for his father leaving. At lunch at my brother's house, he had more helpings than anyone else, and she stared pointedly at him, then looked at me almost smirking, triumphant. She had never liked my only boy – saw him as the obvious favourite because of that uniqueness, and often reacted oddly to people eating.

Being driven about in a car is the one thing that Mother loved best of all. She said she found it restful and once I had begun to take her out regularly on a Sunday, she always complained that I did not take her far enough. My confidence with driving distances, plus the agoraphobia, restricted us to Richmond or Hampton Court, or even Teddington and Hampton Hill. She was always saying what a nervy and sensitive person she was, but never seemed to think that I may have what I call 'funnies' of my own.

Still, the problem of her wishes to travel breaks some of our hearts. Even with her now in a Home, Hayley asked me, only the other day, if we could do something. She would be prepared to pay and take us both on a day trip somewhere. We talk about it often, but get no further with the idea.

There would be steps to climb and Mother can hardly walk. She is incontinent, and I am squeamish. Maybe we could employ one of the Carers on her day off... if it were allowed... if one would agree. Then there is the question of whether I could manage all that arranging. Of course I would at least have taken her further afield in this country on the Sunday runs, were it not for the agoraphobia.

Apart from all that is known of that condition, there is something else which may be peculiar to me. People go on about the beautiful countryside and scenery and sunsets, and I am told that I should enjoy it, but countryside does nothing for me. I look and think, so what? It makes no difference to my life. People have tried to persuade me I am wrong and should try to like it, as if I never had. With places being so much a part of our way of life, our leisure pursuits and educational trips, how could I have escaped it?

The History of Painting slide show which features mostly landscapes, the walks with ramblers – to get company – through bleak local parks, the weekend workshop in a large old house set in deep countryside. And that without a mother to please, whose deep desire was to be taken where I did not want to go.

For sure, I have been in those places more than most people visit what they do not like, and I wonder how it would be if I bullied someone to come and see a Gilbert and Sullivan show or somehow tricked them into attending a philosophy lecture – as my mother manipulated me to sit through a Spiritualist Service – or told them they were fools because they did not like poetry? I have been called a fool sometimes.

For so the nature of some excursions has been cunningly disguised – maybe a car conveniently refusing to go further – and I have ended in a field when I thought I was going to the sea! (I do love the sea.) What if I were to give out invitations to a party and then produce a selection of poems?

The morning glory!

But this too

Can never be my friend.

I read this haiku on one of those tear off calendars. It is by Basho. I keep it, pinned to a magnet on my fridge. Knowing that he would understand me if nobody else does. They don't even know that aspect of it in me – the sense of loneliness and the feeling that this scenery I am supposed to love does not ease that.

And I have many more symptoms of agoraphobia as well. I can be frightened if presented with a new journey, which I really have to make. I am frightened of going to new places and terrified of driving a great distance, especially on motorways. I even feel sick and ill in some places, which are not far away or new to me The black sinking feeling which I have experienced in some Stately Homes does make me question that I may have lived there in a previous life. Going somewhere, especially new or difficult to get to in the evening makes me feel tired. I sometimes wonder whether some of that springs from the days when I was on my own with the children and had no money and no car. I felt I should take them out, particularly in the school holidays, but the thought of getting us all to the bus, then the thought of the cost of the outing, filled me with a disabling heaviness.

The term agoraphobia, like perhaps IBS and ME – and of course dementia – is a blanket term which covers many symptoms and has many causes. Only very recently has someone told me that it can even manifest in a fear of certain groups of people. That has thrown a lot of light, for me, onto my life, for I have tried joining clubs to meet more people. That would have been particularly useful when I embarked on running my business and needed to reach out for more contacts.

Some of these groups have been specifically for single people and I hoped to meet a partner. But I have not always enjoyed them, have felt out of it and odd, and have approached each meeting with a feeling of dread. Strange when I am a social person who attends and runs groups.

Clearly, some mixes of people are as frightening as some places, but knowing that this can be a form of agoraphobia does clear up a puzzle.

Funny, I have never thought of joining a support group for this affliction, or even finding more out about it. Anyway, I am too busy at present sorting out too many puzzles, including that of my mother.

Chapter 22

Today, as I drive home from an all-day philosophy workshop, I think of my agoraphobia and my mother's totally opposite wanderlust. I adored the workshop. The subject was time, and I enjoyed the discussion about what `time` means, and the idea that all time exists. My brain was a jangle with rare intellectual fulfilment.

Mother wants to travel, and I do not know whether that is an escape, or a search for more in life. Travel to me is in the mind, and maybe her search will one day lead her to the same conclusions. I think of Mother's looming ninetieth birthday and the fact she has never been abroad. Gordon did take her on that trip to Calais, when she was in her early seventies and he was able to take her by himself. The thought of the ninetieth brings back memories of the eightieth birthday, when we had a family party at Victor's home, and as she cut the cake, she winged. 'I haven't been round the world. I want to go round the world.' I could almost hear the little girl grizzle of, 'I don't want to be eighty.'

What are we going to do with her next big birthday? Will she last until we have made a plan to get her to France, to Paris? Can I take her somewhere in my car? And why have I not been able to take her far?

My agoraphobia is particularly getting to me, today as I drive home from the philosophy workshop, since a woman in the group told me that she had to leave the class a bit early because she is singing tonight in Mozart's Requiem, which I adore, and have never heard performed live.

Again, the feeling of exhaustion spreads over me as I near home and think of all I would have to do to get to the woman's concert. I would need to eat, get ready, look up the route, find the way, and then somewhere to park.

Mavis, the singer, has a son who has Cerebral Palsy, and we discussed the vicissitudes of any kind of caring. She told me that, every year, she has to fill out, one more time, forms to apply for her son's benefits, and the forms always ask if he still has disabilities.

'I feel like saying no,' she said. 'I feel like saying, no, he suddenly became normal.'

'I know,' I said, 'it is the same with my mother's taxi card. You know you can get this card which gives you cheaper taxi rides, if you can't walk? I got hers five years ago, and every year I had to fill in the forms again. I felt they were expecting me to write back saying I don't want it. Just like you, I often felt like writing that Mother was suddenly able to run up the road.'

So I have enjoyed my Saturday, a wonderful philosophy lecture, meeting Mavis and having a laugh, but the visit to see Mother tomorrow, and the missed Mozart tonight make me feel low.

*

'Lux aeterna in perpettuum' – the words of the Requiem.. I would like to bring eternal light to my mother, I think as I sit with her the next day. She is nagging me about the shop again. Have I been to the old shop lately? Have I been to see 'Mum,' and if not, then I am terrible not to have done so. 'She was good to you,' she suddenly blurts out. Well, I don't remember that! I was only ten when she died, and I remember very little except that I had arguments with her when she would not have it that I had already had ten Christmases when I was only nine, not hearing what I said about having had one when I was nought.

'Will you take me to the shop now? Mother asks.

'It's a long way away,' I say gently.

'No it isn't. It's only up the road. You, know, opposite the old pub.' I look at her and remember when she was just forty, soon after her mother had died. I recall her older brother, Ernest, coming to our house in Essex, and her bursting into tears as soon as she saw him. Even then I knew it was to do with some hankering for the past, a past which had not been good, but held more future and more hope than now, with the children and domesticity. I was not aware of her having a frequent, never mind loving or helpful, relationship with her brother.

Then I recall a day, year's later. I had a baby by then and my father had taken my mother, me, my husband and the baby to visit Aunty Nellie in the East End of London, to show the new baby to her. Aunty Nellie still lived in Forest Gate, where she had always lived and where the little Nellie used to run with her bags on the tram. It was not far from Leytonstone, where the shop had been.

As we set off home, my mother turned to Dad and said, 'I don't want to go near the old shop today.' I suppose it was too painful for her to see it again, the first time since her mother had lived there and the first time since her mother had died, but he drove us past it anyway.

'You can take me, can't you?' she is asking. 'You have your car.'

You know I have a car, you went out in it every week until recently I say to her silently. I look at her face and think of all the nastiness behind it, all the pain that must sit behind that mask.

Once, when we were out, my old Mini broke down, and she had to sit it out with me as we waited for the AA man to come.

'And after you paid all that money for it,' she smirked, and I knew what she was actually saying, I had been done.

Since the Mini had only cost £500, I thought at the time that my mother does give me a few laughs really.

But she did think that was a lot of money, and I believed the intension was to rub in the fact that I am a pushover – as well as poor because I am not worthy of any man really caring for me and providing me with a reliable car. In other words, I am as she was, and she is gloating over my pain, making her forget her own.

I wonder if, like she thinks if you are rich you buy a lovely house that stays lovely without the disruption of decorators or builders, she also imagines wealth buys you a car which never breaks down.

'No,' I say now. 'I can't take you to the shop, I don't know the way.'

Beautiful Dreamer

Chapter 23

So now here we are, it is the ninetieth birthday, and I get to Churchfield House early to check that everything is ready. I walk in to be greeted by the usual urine whiff, but soon cheer up when I see the table is all set in the conservatory. I am overwhelmed by the generosity as I see that the Home has given us a free birthday cake as well as providing a tea at a ridiculously low cost.

Some of the relatives have whinged about the one pound seven-five per head I have asked for, saying why do we need to eat at all. The party is being held between lunch and evening meal time, but it is Mother's ninetieth and she has few pleasures in life. And surely, most social occasions are centred round a meal? Although I tried saying that, nothing changed. They did not listen to me.

What else was there to do for us but eat?

Bring on the dancing girls?

(As long as one of them is me!)

I walk through the building to check with the cook on how the preparations are going, and then I go in to greet Mother on her special day.

The family start arriving, and I am pleased to see that most of them have managed to come even from great distances.

Mother has nine grandchildren, most with partners, and some with children of their own. Mother looks good today. Her hair is white and fluffy, and she has a clean blue dress on that matches her eyes, and she is wearing her gold cross.

The Carers told me recently that my mother gets them to change her clothes two or three times a day, but I cannot help thinking, that cleanliness is not the only reason. I am sure it is more to do with control – she will have people to dress her every day now, well at least that dream has come true for her, she always wanted me to dress her. But maybe they don`t consult her.
Perhaps it provides some small sense of control, to ask for a different dress later on, then to ask for a second time? Well, how much power do any of these residents have left over their lives?

Mother sits at the table in her wheelchair and, as well as the family, I have invited Grace and her husband, both leading healers of the church Mother used to attend. I remember again how the only things Mother ever told me about that church was the laying on of hands and the giving of messages, and that jogs my memory with something I had forgotten.

Once, Mother attended a Quaker church. I asked her at the time how she had liked it, knowing that the services were held in complete silence, with nobody speaking at all and I couldn't see her enjoying that.

'But they don't half jaw when they go into the other room for tea,' she told me. She did have her moments of humour, and how I have always wished there had been more.

We start the present opening and Mother actually seems grateful, even pleased with her gifts. Most of all she loves the gold watch given to her by Gordon, looking at it again and again, and saying repeatedly how lovely it is. I notice that several times during the afternoon she looks down at it again and touches it. Is gold the sign of being loved, something valuable, to make you feel valued yourself, I wonder.
Refreshing memories wash over me as I remember other times when she has been well behaved and, even shone.

In the early days when I came out of that short second marriage and into my present house, I was without a job, so I tried to run my own business. It was a small private Adult Education venture, where I hoped to teach at least two weekly classes and arrange one-off talks. I arranged speakers on a wide variety of subjects including, a landscape archaeologist, a historian, a spiritual healer, a real American Indian, a nutritionist, a jeweller, and a 'colour' lady. My son led some sessions on First World War Poetry.

The Archaeologist obviously had to take us out into the country, and there were also some interesting history walks around Richmond and Kingston. Once, to augment the business, I advertised in a local paper and asked people to join me in Pembroke Lodge, in Richmond Park, to have lunch and discuss my plans. It was a Sunday, and so I took Mother along to the meeting.

Unfortunately, not many came along, in fact there were not many more than my usual faithful band. The business did indeed flounder in the end as there was too much work for virtually no return, and I felt as though I were trying to make a living out of a handful of friends.

Mother had been ready when I picked her up that day, and she looked very clean and tidy. The weather was quite fresh and she had on a clean white beret. At the end of the day, I told her that she had looked very nice and she turned to me and said that she had not wanted to let me down. She had let me down on many other occasions, as I recalled with pain how as a child I went out with friends who were so prettily dressed – and I was not – but maybe she would have liked not to let me down then, well part of her at least.

'You did very well to come,' I said. 'You did not know how many people could be there. You were very brave.' Mother looked at me in absolute amazement. It was as though she had never received praise, and I thought at the time, is your problem just that you have never had any positive reinforcement?

There were other times too, when she was to be admired, like when she managed to fix her own radio battery, instead of waiting for one of us to come and do it for her.

'I didn't want it to beat me,' she said, and I wondered at the ambivalence in any human being, and also how much that resourcefulness had been 'beaten' out of her – the back bashing, the putting down of the brothers, Dad laughing at her piano playing and saying `what could you do?` at the suggestion of her finding a job.

Suddenly I remember a Christmas a decade or two ago.
Mother actually played a quiz game with my children and her pride when she knew some of the answers, especially those about Hampton Court and Henry VIII, was magical.

How I wish we had that quiz game for her now.

The Home cannot prevent the other residents coming into the conservatory, so they wander in and wander out, mingling with the family. One old man, Bernard, sits at the table throughout, and enjoys speaking to some of the family. The Alice in Wonderland 'playing card' lady walks in, as straight as a board, her whole bearing menacing, and she seems almost propelled by some force that drives her as she barges towards first one child, then another. Hayley's young Freddy is terrified.

People are beginning to leave, and all I can think about is the joy of seeing my mother looking so serene at her special birthday party. Hayley turns to me. 'You know, every week when I put down the telephone phone after calling Nanny, I wonder if that will be the last time I will speak to her; but today I can see us all sitting here for the centenary.'

Then I wonder if her peaceful contentment today has anything to do with her spiritual healer sitting by her side and whether she is sending her positive vibes or something.

When everyone has finally gone, I spend five minutes alone with Mother to bridge the gap.

'How do you feel about your ninetieth birthday? I ask.

'I wish I had travelled more, seen the world a bit more.'
The sad look on her face rings in my ears as it has done for over fifty years.

Why didn't you go? I ask softly.

'I didn't know how to go about it,' she says sadly.

Chapter 24

As I drive home, I wonder at this 'not knowing how to go about it.' My mother has always said that she is inadequate, and I partly accepted that, but also wondered if she was like that because she was told so, had it instilled into her from a young age. I know more than one person who has been told as a child that they were no good or could not do things, and they have grown up to fulfil those roles, and didn't my mother grow up with the name of 'silly little Nellie'?

Mother has always hated her name, saying that 'Nell' or 'Nellie' sounded like an old sheep dog. Of course her 'posh' aunt was Nellie, and people did shorten names in those days.
One of my great grandmother Charlotte's older daughters was named after her, but was always known as 'Lottie,' but I wonder if my mother would have felt better about herself if she had been called by her real name, Eleanor? It was more 'noble' sounding, and I am now beginning to think more about something I should have considered years ago.

Mother has always claimed that she comes from the aristocracy, the constant chorus of my childhood days being, 'we may be poor but we are not common.' A lady would not have to know how to `go about things`, would she? She would have had her travel arrangements made for her.

My mother has a high, narrow, somewhat bumpy, nose which she has always claimed to be a sign of aristocracy.
She doesn't like it, and one of her dreams on winning the pools, would have been to get a new nose. Maybe her fine pencil drawings of ladies with high cheek bones are her idea of noble women, but with luckier noses. Mother claims that she comes from the Percy line and the Dukes of Northumberland. Her grandfather was a Peircey but she said that derived from Percy.

The story she tells is that her grandfather was cut off from his family and his inheritance, because he married a girl who was beneath his station. I don't think the lowest class, just not as 'posh,' or as high up the society ladder as them, and in marrying he was cut off without a penny.

One never knows how much of this is a family fable, but from my great aunts and even from my father I was told that my great-grandfather was an artist and a very clever man. He went to The Westminster School and was made a Freeman of the City of London. He designed or made one of the fountains in the capital. He was reported to be good at mathematics and to hold poetry readings in his home.

Most of my children are mathematicians and I hold literary meetings in my home, so the interests in these subjects do run through the family. Both he and one of his sons are reputed to have appeared on stage in Royal Command Performances, drawing quick sketches while telling jokes at the same time. Sadly both he and that particular son died in their thirties of a brain haemorrhage.

George and Charlotte had many children, and I have heard tales of how she married at sixteen and sewed all her own trousseau. She had twenty pregnancies, not all resulting in long living children, or even a live baby. Poor Charlotte, widowed so young, lived to a great age and was blind at the end, and my mother can remember her calling her ` my little Nellie.'

Orphaned and cut off from what might have been, it fell to the older ones to support the family, and my grandmother and two of the older girls took on a shop. It is only since my mother's death that I have begun looking into my grandmother`s family history, or rather I managed to find a Percy who has done forty years of research into the family.

He is a Piercy but explained that anyone called Percy, Piercy or Peircey is definitely descended from the Percys who came from France. He also said something to me that I had never known, that to own a shop in those days, as the aunties and later my grandmother did, was a sign of comparative wealth compared with the poverty and lower class that I had associated with being a shop keeper.

Clearly my great-grandfather was a man of substance, because records show that he insisted on the correct spelling of his surname, He would not have been able to do that without the education and inner strength of having been born into money and position. I wonder how much deeply inherited bitterness there has been inborn into some of my family – a deep rooted gene memory of being cut off from one's roots and fortunes.

I knew some of the aunties like Nellie, and Amy whose husband died so young leaving her broken hearted, and I knew of Felix who had a twirly, waxed, moustache and whose wife I was told had cut her own throat after cleaning the house thoroughly from top to bottom. (Secretly, I have always thought that I might cut my throat if I cleaned that much.) The aunt `Lottie` lived in Scotland and I never met her. Any more of Charlotte's children either lived too far, were dead, or not interested.

The youngest of those children I did know about, Leonard, and he was an artist, a painter. My brother and I stayed with his wife and daughter when our sister was born. I have regular contact with the daughter, Barbara, and she informs me that they were 'a horrible family.' I think she means my grandmother, Nellie, and Amy, and she also told me that Amy's son married a Jew, and nobody would visit her except for Barbara's mother and one other.

Whatever the cause, this was clearly an ailing family, and I wonder if it were all to do with fallen fortunes, or was there another cause? I can certainly see that as the root of my mother's behaviour, in her belief that she was born for better things. Of course, she also had her father, Ernest, and also Charlotte's blood running through her veins. Neither of these came from nobility, but Mother's father was middle class, and I know that he came from a family who could afford help in the home. We all inherit different bits of our past, one sibling perhaps more like his parental side, and another leaning more to the maternal line, but I am beginning to see some light shining on my mother's inability to look after her children as well as our friends' mothers did.

My mother's father, Ernest, was one of a large family whose mother died when they were young. The children's father did indeed leave the care of his children to paid help and Mother told me that she thinks the Carers 'siphoned' some of the money away, the children were not fed properly, and hence Ernest's early death, and what was called his 'nervous debility.' I often wonder whether Jack's paid helpers took the money for my mother's shoes and bought cheaper ones.

What malaise lurked in that household? Why did Jack – a mother in the early twentieth century – have to 'go in the shop,' and leave her children? She did have a husband to support them while they were young. In some of the photographs of my grandmother she looks quite hard, and my young brother says he remembers her like that, looking hard, even though she died when he was two. And although she so often looking scared or pleading, my mother has that same expression at times, especially when abusing me or refusing to put herself out. What goblins were around that made a woman leave her eighteen month old baby in the bath?

Maybe Grandmother had good reason to be sour faced, what with lost birth right and a nervy husband who did not provide, but more and more I think that what ailed her – and whatever led her to it – has ricocheted down the years to my mother and me, crippling us both. An interesting word when you consider that we never knew Jack without crutches. There was nothing wrong with her as far as I know, but she could not walk because she was overweight and had bad legs, and of course there was the broken arm.

It is strange the way my mother talks constantly of her mother dressing her in brown velvet, of brushing her lovely auburn hair and tying it with a brown velvet bow, rather like music being 'one fine day,' and History nothing but Henry VIII and his wives. The hair and the bow seem to be the only examples of real maternal care she ever talks of. The private school cannot be counted since Mother was not happy there, and I sometimes wonder if the velvet bow is not a case of the lady protesting too much. My mother has always had a thing about what she calls `favourites`, asking whenever she meets a family with children, 'who is the favourite?` She goes on at me so much about who she thinks I favour that I wonder who was the favourite in her household?

She has never, to put it mildly, had any affection for my son, other than to ask him when he was three if he would take her out in his car when he grew up! She particularly seemed to be almost in distress when she saw him eating, always saying that he ate too much. One day, I told her that experts were now saying that a boy of fourteen needs more food than his father, and she said that in her day the boys always got the larger portion, 'not like us poor girls.' That statement made me wonder if she were landing on my son's head all the anger she had experienced from her childhood, a world where boys were more important.

Surely in those days, way beyond and even to some degree now, it was in the air that men were better. When my sister had her first baby and it was a boy, just as my mother had a boy first, she asked Valerie if she didn't feel kind of special because she had produced a male and yet, in the family she came from, she was the only one to be sent to private school. Only near the end of her life did she say that she had often wondered if the boys minded. Did that mean that she thought they had reason to 'put her down'?

Certainly, she was put down and cannot have thought herself to be singled out with favours since she was called 'silly little Nellie' and did all the chores behind the shop. And surely a person who was favoured would not have taken the putting down anyway?

My uncles could well have inherited some chips on their shoulders because of the fortune they might have been born into, not to mention the heavy burden it must be on any male to know that they are 'the best,' and have that to live up to.

Ernest was put out at having younger siblings after ten years on his own. He left home early, marrying a woman a lot older than himself, and Mother says it was because the shop was next to a fish and chip place and he could never get rid of the smell of fish on his clothes, but maybe it was also because of some malaise hanging over the place.

For men with their noses born out joint, such resentment would surely have been reinforced by having a mother who was to be reckoned with. She was not a typical woman of her time, owning her own shop, working, and would not have been a figure to treat shabbily, not as would be the norm in the general experience of those boys. How tough to be in a household where the dominant person is a woman. Impossible to bear when all around you were women who could be a victim for any man, so making him the big, strong and important one.

What other reason could there be for treating my mother as they did? There was this small woman in the same household who could be punished for the feelings of self-doubt or inadequacy resulting from having the mother they did.

Albert stayed in the shop forever, even when married, and what he did to my father can have no explanation, for me, other than that this destruction of his sister had to go on. He somehow bullied my father to go and work for the family business, so condemning my dad to a lifetime as a lowly paid shop manager, and my mother and her children to a life of poverty. The punishing of his sister for his mother's strength must have come from a very deep need, that lasted and spread to his treatment of me.

In a way, I was a bigger threat, because I was clever. was capable. He could never have claimed me to be inadequate. It was as though Snow White's stepmother had got rid of the girl only to find there was another girl, another threat. Albert's strong mother was a threat to his manhood.
He created a new reality in disempowering his sister, then he found himself faced with yet another strong woman.

*

And so the day little Nellie reaches ninety, her daughter arrives at new clues to her mother's sorrow. Her lack, a born lady's ease and privilege. A mother soured by so much, and a brother who had to make her bottom of the pecking order – so that it would not be him. She did not like men, and that is certainly of her brothers doing. She was ambivalent, speaking of them with love or pride, and missing them at times. She used Albert too, going to him with problems and asking for money, but every now and again whenever she said he ought to help her more, she would spit bitterly that, after all, it was he who had 'got Dad into this awful job.'

Of her sons she could speak nothing but good. Her daughters' husbands, boyfriends, sons or sons-in-law were nearly always maligned.

She certainly hated my son more than most, probably because he is the only boy in a family of four, and she assumed he would be the 'favourite' from the minute he was born, coming to see me the next day with her cries of 'where are the girlies?' That whining voice told me it all: that the two, poor, older sisters were now going to have their noses put out of joint.' where are the little girlies?'

All his childhood, she nagged me non-stop , that he was spoilt, and it was a constant barrage of attack going on for most of any visits. If I tried to defend myself, to deny the charge, she would say, 'oh, you just can't see it.' One time she was so vindictive to him that I threw her out of the house.

I marched her to the front door, opened it, pushed her out and closed it. All was quiet for a whole two weeks, before she telephoned and asked in a very polite, posh, put-on voice if she could `come to` my house.

When she first saw me nursing him she whined, 'oh, don't have any more babies,' and I knew it was nothing to do with care for me, thought for my finances, my lifestyle, or some possible future career, or even for my health. It was because she wanted to be my baby. I did have one more, another girl, and she did become my mother's favourite, but not even for her would my mother 'put herself out.' Once Imogen kept asking her nanny to read her a particularly long story and Mother refused, continuing to refuse until the child gave up.

My poor children eventually found it easier to keep out of the way, and they had to play, do homework or whatever, and I kept my mother with me in one room. Those Sundays while they were still young and before I was free to take her out in a car, saw indoors the ritual of the coffee, the lunch, the tea.
Then there would be the walk to the bus stop with a drink in a pub on the way. We sometimes set off on this last stage too early, and some pubs were still closed, and to an onlooker it could have looked like we were on a pub crawl!

Yes, there were moments to laugh at, like one of the Sundays when I had cooked a roast dinner. It was at a time when my personal life had hit one of its lows, and I guess coping with Mother while deeply depressed would have traumatised anyone. So, in clearing the meal, I was doing my usual saving of bits, slivers of cold meat from the plates, leftover vegetables into plastic pots and so on. I even saved the unused gravy, which could be put into tomorrow's stew.

There stood the gravy jug and next to it the milk jug. Mother liked her tea from a teapot and milk in a jug, as any lady's maid would provide! The milk could go back into the milk bottle, except that it was the gravy I poured in there. Never mind, I thought, after all, it was a fairly full bottle of milk, and there was not too much gravy left, so I made teas and coffees for everyone for the rest of the day and nobody noticed.

Today, here on her ninetieth birthday, Mother has not given us one laugh, but at least I am a little way on in my search to what ails her, and one could almost laugh hysterically with relief to see her for once at peace. But it would be nice to smile so I think I'll pretend to myself that we played a quiz game today.

Then I recall something that was awful at the time, but which does now makes me smile. It was one time when the children were young and Mother was having lunch with me, I found myself cooking something different for everybody. The girls did not eat much and were picky anyway, Rafe was still a baby, and Mother I knew would expect to be given a treat.

First I brought in small plates for Anna and Hayley with a couple of chipolata sausages on one and fish fingers on the other. My mother did not know it, but her feast was still cooking, eggs with bacon and tomatoes. Next I came in with a boiled egg for Rafe, and from Mother it was 'ooh's and ah's' and 'oh, he's the king, he's the king.' I wondered if she was somewhat abashed when her large plateful came in. But what was that all about? A boiled egg?

Perhaps it was something to do with the fact that it looked more than two little sausages? Or was an egg in an egg cup raised high, like a present carried on a cushion to the king on his throne. The lovely girl set up above the throne, and made even higher with a crown on her head. Now I remember how she called the 'rich and the posh,' the 'high-ups.'

Chapter 25

I think of monsters as I walk towards my mother today, seated in her usual corner. She is a monster in my life, and that is how she looks today. The new teeth have arrived from the dentist, and she looks like some caricature of a monster.

Mother's false teeth. She had all her teeth taken out at the age of twenty, having been told it would be easier. When I was a teenager, she used to have a midday rest on my bed and it seems she took her teeth out for sometimes at night, as I went to set the alarm on my clock on the bedside table, there were Mother's teeth – grinning at me.

Today she growls. 'These teeth don't fit.' The bottom set of teeth stick out as if she were purposely pushing her bottom jaw out. I can't believe that any dentist could get it so badly wrong. Yet more for me to sort out, I think. Yes, her new bottom teeth stick out, it seems, in front of the top teeth like some kind of a dog, perhaps a bull dog.

Funny I should think of a dog, because when I had all the children at home, the house to run, and was studying for my degree, she was always picking on this and that, and it felt like I had a little dog snapping at my heels. Somehow it seemed to be worse to bear when I was busy, and she seemed to hate me being busy, presumably because it meant that I was too busy to give her my sole attention. It was particularly hectic when the children had boyfriends or just school friends around. I would be cooking for at least eight people – a regular event and one which I enjoyed. She would be there going on and, yes, it did feel as though she were snapping at my heels like a little dog. Why did I have to do so much? Why couldn't they be at their friends' houses?

Or was the needling me really fuelled by the fact that she felt guilty because she had never worked as I did?

I actually enjoyed having all the family for a meal and it needled me that she was rubbing it in how downtrodden I was. I remember leaving her in the shops when I had some of the children with me, and perhaps they had whined for sweets and toys, or perhaps I had a hard time trying to find them new clothes or shoes at a price I could afford. As I left her and looked back to wave goodbye she would be standing square on looking at me, almost accusingly, but pityingly, as if she were saying, 'look at you, the poor wife, who has no time for treats for yourself because you have all these children.'

I look at my mother today, thinking of all she used to say to me. Why didn't I take myself right off out of it, she used to say when I was doing all that cooking. What mother would leave her children to fend for themselves? Get myself off out of it — like you did? That is what I should have replied. Going to Worthing for days on your own? Leaving me to look after everything?

These terrible teeth. She has waited long enough for the first set, which did not fit and now we get monstrosities Presumably they pleased the dentist when he came to see her, but maybe he was half blind and did his work by feel. I tell the Carers the teeth must go back, and the dentist will have to have another go, even if it takes another six months.
Poor Mother, I remember her telling me, a few years before she came into Residential Care, that a dentist had told her teeth were not fitting because her gums were crumbling. Yet another small heartbreak. Part of her decaying already.

A bit like when I told Anna, aged six, that Nanny`s hair was dyed, and she thought I meant `died'. Dying in stages.

It is the chiropodist visit today and, as I sit with Mother waiting her turn, I watch the residents whom I have come to know well. There is Iris who has worked all her life in a children's nursery, and now she thinks all the old ladies and men are her charges. 'She won't eat her dinner today,' she tells a Carer. 'His mother hasn't come for him,' she says to me, pointing to Bernard and looking very anxious.

May sits agitated as always. She has to get home. How are they all going to cope without her at home? The train must come soon. 'You do not want to ride on trains too late in the day,' she warns. 'There are some nasty people, some nasty things happening on trains.'

Bernard comes up to me and asks is it Sunday, and has he been to Mass this morning. He reads the Daily Telegraph and sometimes I pinch the crossword from him as that is the only one

I can do, and I can no longer afford newspapers. He used to do that crossword too but not anymore.

Once he invited me to his room, and I went briefly while Mother was been taken to the toilet. He had a computer switched on, and he told me that he had lived and worked abroad. He went on to tell me about his son who lives and works on the same place and earns too much money there to be able to come back and live near his Dad, or even to come over from time to time. Bernard said he totally understands and accepts that. 'Come and see me again,' he said.

We are taken up in the lift, Mother in her wheelchair, and we sit while the chiropodist finishes the client before Mother. Then she begins on Mother's feet, beginning with the one with the worst twisted big toe. It comes to me what some of my spiritual books say about the body's ills. Problems with the feet and walking are claimed to be an indication of the lack of inner growth, since the feet are literally for going forward.

I think of the Chinese women who have their feet bound and how the stunting of their physical ability to walk may have blighted their personal development. Interestingly, I have also read that women who undergo the very worst form of female circumcision can hardly walk. So any form of disempowerment of women will reach beyond to all parts of their lives.

What came first, the feet or the crippled personality? Did whatever happened to my mother's growth manifest itself in the twisted toes?

'What can be done?' I ask, and the chiropodist explains that all she can do for most of the old people is make their feet more comfortable, prevent toe nails from getting too long and remove any hard skin. That reminds me that Mother had a slight fall recently. She fell when she tried to get out of bed in the night to use the commode. She told me later that the floor was very slippery.

'Would it be a good idea for her to wear socks in bed?' I ask the chiropodist, after explaining about the fall. 'Those ones with the grips underneath,' I suggest.

'They would probably make her feet too hot,' the woman replies, but she promises to send me a catalogue of footwear for difficult feet, just in case there are some 'grippy,' but thin, socks I could order.

I feel that we are both looking with amazement at Mother's feet, with the big toe at right angles across the other ones.
'Could it have been caused by ill-fitting shoes? I ask.

'Well, it is mostly genetic,' she says, so I show her my feet.
Already my big toe points slightly inwards.
'Is there anything I can do to stop them getting worse, getting like Mother's?'
'No, it's genetic. But don't worry, it does become watered down.'

So, the inherited bad feet get better with each generation, I think. I was told the beautiful figure was genetic . Will that be 'watered down' too?

What do I inherit from the Percy family – bitterness, aristocratic inadequacy? Or of the finer side of nobility?

I go back with Mother to her usual seat, and prepare for the complaints when I am ready to leave. Then I notice a new resident. She has presumably brought her own tall backed chair with her, and it looks like a throne. I am reminded of a queen sitting on a throne, and the egg in its egg cup which made my mother call my little boy a `king`.

This woman is upright and has her hair piled high into a bun on the top of her head. She wears chains and bracelets, and rings in heavy gold. 'Who is that? I ask Mother's Key Worker when she brings in the coffee.

'That is Prunella. She lived in India all her married life, and her husband must have held quite a high position because she keeps saying that he was the British Empire. Maybe he was an ambassador or something? She behaves like she thinks that she is some kind of empress, if you ask me.

'Does she believe she is holding some kind of court here? Are we all her servants?` I ask.

'Probably,' laughs the Carer.

Well, at least someone has found a way of re-writing the script, and a way to be happy here. I drink my coffee quickly as I suddenly remember I have reading to do for my literature class. I pick up my bag and get away smartly, ignoring the protests. On the way out, I bump into Bernard. 'How are you today?' I smile at him.

'I am lost and alone,' he says.

I don't know what to say. His son never visits and he is still a clever man but has lost his memory. I can feel a real reaching out of someone's soul, but I don't know how to touch it.

I drive home thinking of the different ways of coping that the residents have discovered, the ways that they have created realities that are better than the stark truth, which is living in a Retirement Home with nothing to look forward to but death.

Iris believes she is still working with children, May believes she is a much younger woman, with a family at home waiting for her return, and now Prunella is still 'queening' it as though she still lives a very different lifestyle in India and has plenty of servants around her.

Yet Iris is always worried, worried about her children, and May is constantly agitated about whether she is going to catch the train in time before it is too late. What did happen to her once, I wonder, what was so 'nasty' on the train? At least Prunella's created reality world is a happy one.

It is only Bernard who faces the truth of his situation and is miserable about the here and now. What he tells me is true of them all – and perhaps of many of us – when he says he is lost and alone.

As I arrive home and let myself into the house, I find myself thinking about Prunella's jewellery. There is something that interests me about women and their adornments. Mother has broken her cross and she seems now to be envying other people's necklaces and brooches. Again I find myself back to my theme of what ails the demented female, and the need for jewellery as part of what I have already seen - the desire to still look glamorous. That desire to look like a cherished woman, as well as other things, requires being seen to have been given valuable gifts?

I decide I must call Sylvia, as I make my cup of Ayur Vedic tea. This is one prescribed by the meditation world for my body type, which is prone to anxiety. I must try to get my mother some new baubles, but I must ring Sylvia. She comes to my creative writing group, and is my greatest companion, often coming out with me and Mother. We really must get my mother to the shops and maybe buy a new cross and chain, but before I can telephone Sylvia, I get a call from the Home. Mother has had another fall.

Putting he phone down and wondering what to do, something else in the day comes back to me. Mother`s appearance with the terrible new teeth which made her look like some kind of dog, is so sad because she always said that `Nellie` sounded like and old sheep dog.

Dogs. Mother snapping at my heels like a nasty, snappy, biting little dog.

Albert once told me he would give me a dog`s life.

Valerie was very little and making a mess with her food.

If she was young enough to be eating so messily, I must have been still a young child myself. Yet he said to me that, if I did not look after her, he would give me a dog`s life.

Chapter 26

Mother's Social Worker whilst she was in the community was Ann Wright, and she was always talking about my mother's 'anxiety.' She spoke of this as if it were the only personality problem that ailed Mother, and was the cause of all her ills, but I always maintained that I did not see anxiety as the main issue that needed to be dealt with. I suppose anxiety Would cause constant discomfort, but how could it explain her treatment of me? Her seeming gloating when she needles me? Or why I was treated so differently to all my siblings?

I too was sent to stay with Auntie Nellie, every year of my childhood, and like little Nellie I went, but not just for a few days, I was sent there for the whole of the summer holidays, and was the only one of all mother's children to do that. When challenged on this, Mother would say that she felt that she could not give me much and I would have a better time with Aunty Nellie. So I wondered why she did not want her other three children to have a 'better time' too.

At Nellie's in Forest Gate, I got lemonade and comics, but there were no children to play with.

Auntie Nellie was a snob and I found it immeasurably painful when she and her stepdaughter jeered at my poor clothes and – worse – made fun of my mother's appearance. She and Freda were nasty about my mother in general – for not being a good housewife, for not keeping her children clean and tidy, and when I arrived for my six week stay, they would open my suitcase and take out each item in turn, hold it up, and laugh. No doubt it was a bag of rags.

Nellie sat looking out of the window at the neighbours and was particularly scathing of anything sexual. She must have looked out of her bedroom window too because she said more than once that the young couple opposite ought to draw their curtains better and what they got up to showed bad breeding. She had married late and I wonder if she had had sex at all. She certainly had little knowledge of that side of life since I once heard her ask a friend just what exactly was meant by a ` breech birth`.

Her residential road was full of little shops including a greengrocer, butcher – all basic provisions were on her doorstep.. It also had a fish and chip shop and an off licence: She went shopping most days, but as she got older she sent me to do it. I took my lemonade and Tizer bottles back and you were given three-pence for each bottle in those days, which went towards my next bottle of fizz. I also bought the whiskey which Nellie took for her arthritis and kept secret from the step-children she lived with.

She used to put the paper bag the bottle came in on the fire saying, 'burn the evidence.' Since then, I have wondered what she did to hide the evidence of the bottle. After shopping one day I told her that I had see a man wearing make-up, and she said he was a 'silly arse.'

It was quite disrupting, been sent to Nellie's every summer, and I think, while I was there, my family must have gone on holiday without me. It seemed to me that we had just a few seaside holidays but, when I said that to Mother much later she said, 'oh no, Dad took us away every year.' Every time I left home I sobbed for my family, but every time I left Auntie Nellie's I sobbed for her too.

I remember it was a worrying time, the summer I went after I had passed to go to the grammar school. By the time I got home, the new term was nearly upon us, and nothing had been done about my uniform. It took my coming back and pressing my mother to get things moving.

Most of all I was heartbroken at missing six whole weeks when my baby brother had not long been born. Six weeks is an enormous amount of time with a new baby. He had changed and I felt I had missed so much. It was quite cosy with Auntie Nellie, and I had my fizz and my comics, but her two step-children were more my mother's age. They were called Freda and Olly, named after his father, and both worked all week. Auntie Freda took me out for days at the weekend to cinemas and parks, and even 'posh teas' with her friends.

There were few children to play with, if any. I once went out onto the street and joined the gang who played out there, but the only activity seemed to be fighting so I never went again. Nellie's neighbour had a child who visited once and I was invited in to see a television for the first time. That was a treat, so I guess I was getting the 'better time' that my mother talked of.

Another neighbour used to let me play in her garden, and hidden among the flowers were a little stone rabbit and a stone tortoise, which have stayed in my mind forever. It was a cosy time with my Aunty, I could draw and read, and both Nellie and Freda played 'consequences' with me – that being even more fun when one of Freda's friends came to join in.

What I loved most was when Auntie Nellie and I sat and listened to the radio, especially when it was 'Mrs Dale's Diary.' That programme was on the radio at elevenses time and sometimes Auntie had made me some bread pudding which I still enjoy, and make it to this day.

That cosy time, that ritual, that comfort zone, is something that I have always wanted to continue, and I did it with my young brother. When I was about fourteen, my mother left me to look after my little brother while she had a break. Every morning we listened to a radio story and had drinks and a doughnut.

Amy lived quite near to Nellie, and visited her occasionally. She was different, she had inherited less of the nobility I would say, being more a busy, housewifery sort of person. Her husband had died young and, according to Mother, it was a blissfully happy marriage. What I saw was a practical woman who gave me and my sister aprons for Christmas.

Every time we moved house, Amy would come and help my mother get the place in order, putting up and even making the curtains. She also chided my mother and talked about her behind her back for not been a better housewife.

After one move, Amy told me that when she was young, people moved whenever they felt like it, it was easy. Most people rented their homes, and they simply went to the renting place and said they wanted to move. She made it sound like buying a new dress, with none of the traumas that we associate with house moves today. In those days it was just a case of variety and fun.

Right to the present day, Mother speaks fondly of how she remembers Amy holding and cradling her when she was a small child and a bomb fell nearby. But it was Nellie to whom Mother went most often, with the packing up of her things and getting on the tram.

Auntie Amy clearly did not like Gordon. Every Christmas, she would give Victor, Valerie and me a wrapped parcel – albeit aprons for us girls. Our baby brother got a two shilling piece in an envelope. It was no wonder since she had lost her husband early and had only one child.

Amy saw my family more often than Nellie, who was fairly housebound with arthritis and knew only me as I went to stay there. But Amy gossiped and soon after Gordon was born, it seemed, Nellie spent her time telling me he was spoilt. As she had no children I wonder if they were jealous of my mother having so many children already, and after four years even one more – and a boy!

The stays in Forest Gate were bad in some ways, but they were also good. Nellie, as well as Freda, took me out to parks and 'posh' cafés, and she also took me out in hired cars. Nellie had arthritis and only walked painfully with a stick. Once, in the hired car, when we were stationery at a junction, some East End children playing in the street looked in the car window and asked if we were millionaires. I felt indescribably strange.

Nellie had had many boyfriends, according to Mother, including Billy who was the longest lasting and had died suddenly. Mother remembers Nellie crying all day into a multitude of silk handkerchiefs. Billy gave her many beautiful rings and these she gave in her lifetime to her relatives.

Mother got one that had three rows of five diamonds, but she never wore it.

Nellie did get married later, to Olly, but she was a widow when I knew her, and I never heard anyone say much about Olly.

Leonard, the artist, lived very near to Auntie Nellie but we rarely saw him. His daughter Barbara, who was about seven years older than me, did come round often, and one day she told us that Len was planning to visit soon. Auntie Nellie was horrified. 'Oh, no,' she said. 'He'll make my sofa dirty.' She was worried about his 'painty' old clothes messing up her 'posh' front room, and even then I thought that I would be proud to have a brother who was an artist.

My mother was put down by her brothers when quite young. Later, because she was nervous, she did not go out to work so was left to do the 'skivvying' behind the shop.

Whatever needed to be done, she told me – mainly washing up – it would always be 'Nell will do it.' No wonder all my childhood it was, 'Pat will do it.'

Constantly put down, washing up behind the shop, then nearly an unmarried mother, my mother had an indecent number of children and was a sluttish housewife. If they had no tolerance for the 'painty' clothes, it is little wonder that she got the criticism she did. There was never any understanding of the gallivanting and gadding about. Albert's wife told me that they were always getting letters from my mother about her life being all drudgery and bed-making, and my mother told me that the only reply she ever got was a reminder of her 'duty' as wife and Mother.

` Duty, duty, duty,` she spat at me.

Thinking of the snobbery and criticism, the vindictive pin-sticking because somebody got a late little boy, I realised they were indeed a horrible family. My mother should not gallivant.

An artist might dirty the sofa! Was there no largesse – and no fun?

Maybe I should forgive my mother for putting me down, using me as her handmaiden and giving me such a hard time about my son, for what other example did she have, what role model did she have on how to treat a girl? But still, that does not explain the deep unhappiness, or the fear I sometimes see on her face.

And did everyone do what was their duty – for her?

Did anyone?

Does everyone now?

… Beautiful Dreamer

Chapter 27

'Go if you are not going to help me.' This was Mother's comment soon after I got to Churchfield today. I can go if I am not going to take her to her mum. I arrived soon after hearing she has had yet another fall. This has happened twice recently, and both times she had fallen while trying to get to the payphone supplied for residents in the Home.

'Who were you trying to phone? I ask her now.

'Mum.'

Then she talked of how she had to get home, Mum needed her.

'But you can't look after yourself,' I replied.

'Oh, I would be all right at home, I could go up the old High Road. I could nip in and out. I'd be cosy. I could take Mum out in her chair.'

'I must leave promptly at quarter to three,' I say, not wanting to go down the route of Mum not being there, the shop probably not being there, and I could not possibly drive to Leytonstone.

'I have to pick Molly up from school,' I say.

'Oh, do you have to?'

'Yes Mother I do. Anna's Carer has had to go somewhere else.'

'Couldn't she find someone else to pick her up?'

'No,' I say firmly.

'Then, go, if you're not going to help me.' I choose to ignore it. I have a bit of time and I show her some school photographs that Anna has just given me of Gregory and Molly. 'I haven't seen the children in years,' she whines.

'They were here at your birthday party, don't you remember?'

'Here you are, Ellie,' a Carer brings us tea. Mother has been called Ellie in both Homes, and she says she prefers it. I would rather it were Eleanor. The cardboard 'playing card lady' walks towards me and I feel that familiar prickle of fear, although I know she will walk past, at the last minute, when she is almost on top of us.

May is fretting about missing the train, and Bernard comes in holding the newspaper looking lost.

'Can I have the crossword ?' I ask, and he smiles and tells me yet again that his son is far away and can't visit, but that he has no choice because he earns so much money where he is. He wanders away to ask Carers if he has been to Mass, and Mother dunks biscuit in her tea, dropping bits down her cardigan.

I rummage through the books and games shelves and find a box of film star photographs. A quick read tells me that it is a 'game,' where the idea is to show each card in turn and see if the other players can identify the faces. I try it on Mother. I show first this one, then that, but she turns away, her hand over her face, shielding her eyes, something she does a lot, especially when trying not to see Rafe.

'Look,' I persist, and put one of the cards right close to her.

'Kay Kendall.' I say. 'She was in 'Genevieve.' You know how you loved that film, all about old cars and outings.'

'Take it away. Take it away.'
She speaks fiercely, then looks at me and asks softly. 'Will you take me out in your car?'

It is bright day, so I suggest that we sit outside. I help her out on her walking frame to the garden seats, where there are tubs of flowers; and beyond the patio flower beds where an old man is walking up and down.

'It is lovely here for you,' I say.

It's not like home`, says Mother. 'It's not the same as being with somebody of your own.'

'They dress you here,' I remind her, for she has always wanted me to dress her.

On the morning of my first wedding, when she was only fifty, I spent more time dressing her than getting myself ready for my own wedding. I remember the scene so well, and wonder yet again what it is all about. She stood before me as I did up a button, fastened a necklace, flicked her hair into place.

Then, I can see my face clearly, as I looked in the dressing table mirror of my childhood. Weary, slumping at the shoulders, and too tired to do my own makeup. So I went to my wedding with hardly any on at all.

She was fifty and I was twenty. I had been shopping with her for her clothes, and on the day I had to put them on her, choose jewellery, make sure the hat was straight, fix her mother-of- the-bride flower. I did her makeup, hair, everything.

And all the time, she stood before me like a little girl.

The message was clear. ` You may be getting married and leaving home, but you will still be my mummy, won't you?`

Words unspoken, but as clear as a bell.

She really always wanted a lady`s maid to dress her.

Suddenly, the old man falls over. I call a Carer and we both rush over to him. Another person comes out with a wheelchair, so I go back to Mother. She is very quiet.

'I expect it is because I am out here,' she says quietly, meek and sad.

'What?'

'I expect that he fell down, because I was here. Things always go wrong when I am around.'

'What do you mean? I ask again.

'Well, I've always thought I had a jinx, on me.'

'Why on earth do you think that?'

'Well, Mum's arm. I have always believed that was my fault that she broke it.'

'But why ever should you think that?'

'I thought somebody said it, that`s all.'

Yet another example of the guilty feelings, the persecution and conspiracy, I note. Like when she recently tried to `phone her mum`, about going home to her, leaving the Residential Home, and heard a voice saying, ` keep her there.`.

'Tell me about it,' I say. 'Tell me about the time when you were little.'

'I had lots of aunties, but Mum had to go in the shop.'

'What did you do when she was in the shop?'

'I listened to the radio a lot, but I didn't like the dark stairs.'

'What happened on the dark stairs, Mother?'

'Oh I don't know, I was always frightened, that's all.'

'Were you abused? There was total silence before she turned to me, frightened.

'It was uncle Olly..'

'Tell me about it.' At last, at last.

'Well, you see, Auntie Nellie married late in life, but by then I had a lot of nice cosy uncles, and I used to sit on their laps. Then when uncle Olly came along, I sat on his lap too. But I wasn't used to him, and he wasn't one of the cosy uncles I'd always had. I sat on his lap.....

` I think it must have aroused his sexual feelings.' She will say no more, and I have to go.

I drive to pick the children up thinking. So – 'posh' Auntie Nellie – she who looked out of her window and bitched about other people's sexual activity – had a husband who abused young girls. My daughter guessed it years ago. Mother has always denied it, and now I know for certain. I must be near the end of my search. I know that being sexually abused as a child could have caused all my mother's ills.

Things are a bit clearer now, for I have learned some basic psychology on some of the many Adult Education courses I have attended. Sexual abuse is immeasurably damaging for a child, but when the perpetrator is a relative, there are far reaching results. Relatives are meant to be protective, not the opposite, so all normal boundaries have been broken down. The child is likely to grow up with no sense of normal boundaries, and perhaps with no sense of normal behaviour.

Sometimes, when your core self has been invaded, you sometimes have no sense of where you begin and another ends, which is probably why Mother has treated me as if I were her. If I were in some way – because of lack of boundaries, because her pain was so great – just an extension of her, then I could have no needs of my own. So why wouldn't I want to do and be what she needed?

Or is it that children who are abused by a relative grow up with no normal sense of right and wrong, for that has been violated? No wonder Mother thought it perfectly all right for me to drive someone else's car without permission.

I turn into my road remembering the times when Mother's totally amoral attitude has shown itself quite outrageously.

If there were a car on the premises belonging to anyone we knew, my husband, my son, my brother, she would nag me to take her out in it even if I said that I was not insured to drive that particular vehicle, or that the owner had not given permission – or I did not have the right kind of driving licence.

'Just for a little run,' she would argue, and 'it won't hurt for once,' or 'they won't know.'

When we lived in the country near Southend, a relative came all the way by train from the East End of London to help her with the housework. It appears that news had got around that we had a slum of a house, and this relative had come to do a bit of spring cleaning. She knocked on the door, but nobody answered. It had turned out to be a lovely day that morning, so Mother had gone out for the day.

It would not have occurred to her to stay in for someone who had made a long journey to help her. The lack of welcome for her relative would not bother her for, if they were stupid enough to come, then they would be glad she was not in, so they could take themselves off somewhere nice and make the most of the day, instead of doing horrible housework. She would not stay in for anyone, and she would not expect them to have come as it had turned out so fine. In her mind nobody would travel a long way in glorious weather to do housework - what she called `sweeping and banging and doing.'

But to go out when a visitor is expected, surely shows no idea of normal behaviour.

Funny how she got us all doing her housework, the visitor from the East End of London was her brother's mother-in-law. Auntie Amy did it, I have done it; we have all done our share of being Mother's lady`s housemaids.

As I park in the drive I see that my front window will soon be obscured by the untrimmed bushes. I will be getting another letter from the Council soon if I don't trim what is overhanging the `public pathway.' My house is fast becoming to look like that of Sleeping Beauty, and soon I will have to hack my way through with a sword to get to the front door. I put the key in the lock, and before checking the answering machine, I do my pelvic floor exercises.

And I wonder how little Nellie knew what an erection was. The erection she felt when she sat on the lap of that non-cosy uncle!

When people are sexually abused by someone in a position of trust, they can lose the ability to trust. They see all men, or women , as abusers.

If, deep down, we believe abusers are all there is, we attract that to us. And so we attract abusers and marry them. Of course we do.

Chapter 28

We have a new minister at the Unitarian Church, after many months of seeking following the last one leaving. The new Minister is called Vanessa and she is beautiful, and young, certainly as young as my two older daughters. I have known her for a month and already she seems the one person in the world who is most like me, being deeply interested in life, spirituality, people and psychology – as well as make-up, clothes and hair!

The church offers frequent discussion groups, and six- week workshops at least three times a year. These are courses from the Unitarian Movement or devised by the minister. I led one meeting when the last minister was unable to take it one week, and in the period of having no minister, I dreamt up and presented my own series of discussion topics.

So here I am this evening at the beginning of a new session called Life's Journey. The Church Newsletter outlined the course as examining childhood, parents, growing up, relationships, work, hobbies and aspirations, and the aim is for the students to see what they have learned in life, look for patterns, and work out how to move forward.

Trudi, who has become my church friend in the last year, is here and also Betty whom I met at an exercise class. Betty is also a Transcendental Meditator and wanted to try my church courses. The two met at one of my selling parties.

Trudi is just eighty and does the coffee and flowers for the church. She also acts as warden some Sundays, greeting the congregation when they arrive, giving out the hymn books and taking the collection. She also plays bridge, and is learning to play the piano, and visits several housebound old friends in their homes.

I had already met Betty at a meeting for meditators, when I bumped into her at an exercise class. She is over eighty too, and was a hairdresser in her working days. She still does hair for a few friends and particularly for her daughter and granddaughter, who live near her. Having recently been diagnosed as having diabetes, she has a lot of medical checks to keep up with, but still maintains her large garden, sews, and works once a week in a hospital dispensary as a volunteer.

As with many courses, groups and meetings - even work related ones I have noticed - we begin with going round the circle of people and asking those present to say something about themselves: marital status, children, work, hobbies, reasons for joining the course, any or none of these. All the sessions begin with a different question each time, like how you are feeling today, and what was the most significant event of the last week. When I was the leader, two of my 'going around the circle' starters were what is your biggest fantasy, and how do you feel about your name.

I have never known much about Trudi's private life, and in the warm up circle she revealed that she has no children. In the tea break I ask her why.

'Because I have never even kissed a man,' she tells me.

'Do you know why?' I ask.

'Yes, I do, I was sexually abused as child.'

'Do you mind telling me more?' I am stunned by this sudden admission. 'Have you told anyone else?'

'No... well I did tell one friend a few years ago, but she didn't believe me.'

'Why did you tell me, so suddenly?'

'Because you have a kind face,' she replies.

'Do you mind if I tell anyone? The Minister? Even write about it?'

'No.'

Her story is that, years ago, she went to a Guide camp. It was very wet weather and she was made to sleep in her sleeping bag even though her part of the ground was exceptionally wet. She became very ill and was taken into hospital with a rare lung disease. The Guide Captain told her the illness was God's will. She was in hospital for a very long time and was working on a stamp collection to amuse herself, but one day, a nurse cleared away all the stamps by mistake.

Trudi was bitterly upset because she had nothing else to play with, but another nurse told her that there was a young boy patient, who collected stamps and maybe he would share some with her. He had quite a large collection because he had been in hospital for a very long time, so Trudi went off to find the boy in the courtyard where he sat every day. They were both lonely and spent a lot of time together, both glad of the other's company.

However, the next time Trudi's parents came to see her, they were called into see the Matron who told them that she had been looking out of her window onto the courtyard and had witnessed Trudi making disgraceful advances to the boy.

Soon after that, Trudi went home and her father began his regular sexual use of her. The child's mother knew what was going on, but both parents told their daughter that what her father was doing to her was for her own good. She never married or had anything to do with men. Ill health continued to daunt her all her life, ruining her education, and although it was clear that she was highly intelligent she never went as high, as she felt she might have done, in her job.

*

As we sit down for the second half of the evening, I am feeling stunned. My mother was abused, Trudi was abused.
Yet Trudi has not become vindictive or in any obvious way damaged. She has always worked and now lives a full and busy life. So there are different ways of reacting to child abuse, I think. Maybe that is not the sole root of my mother's problems after all, of her Personality Disorder. Was it the bomb falling near her home that caused it? The endless put downs? Was it the lifelong poverty and lack? Maybe one's reaction to anything depends on all sorts of variables, including the personality you are born with. And of course Trudi did not have children with all the limitations to building a life they can bring.

As we leave the church, I see Trudi is being taken home by another eighty year-old, Mary, whom I do not know. 'Listen here,' Trudi is calling to me. 'I'm regretting my education even more now. Guess what Mary does? She and three of her friends have a 'Greek' group. They read books in Greek, and discuss them. Aren't they lucky?'

I drive home thinking that, just as there is more than one way of being affected by child abuse, there are also many ways of being an eighty year-old.

*

Today Vanessa is visiting me, and as I stand at the window hoping she will be able to find her way through the bushes, I hear a knock at the door. She is small, so I have not seen her pass my window. As she comes into my house, we both ask each other where we bought our tops. `Charity shop,` we both say laughing, and commenting that therefore neither of us can hope to find another one like the other`s.

Now as I make coffee, I tell her all about me, since she wanted to know. I speak of my too-young marriage and my widely spaced family of four, of my degree in later years, my second marriage to an abuser and the divorce that followed which, if not illegal, was certainly not conducted in an equitable way. I talk about my mother and my un-fulfilment in every area of my life. I say that I want a lover above everything else. Also that, at the age of eleven, I was sexually abused by my father.

Then I turn to Trudi, and her life story. We talk of the different affects that such abuse can have on children. I confess to her my lifelong depression, and my many and varied attempts to heal it. She finishes her coffee.

'Just one thing,' she says as she stands up to go.

As she pauses, I wonder what it could be. More about the abuse perhaps? How the church can help me? Can she help me with Mother? Could I help with the church flowers or coffee?

'Just one thing,' she hesitates then asks.

'Your hair is so pretty. Where do you get it done?'

*

Do I tell Mother about Vanessa's comments about my hair?

I laugh to myself after the Minister has gone and return to my bedroom to write my weekly letter to Imogen. She is expecting her first baby now and I do not feel that I give her enough of my time. Classes, writing, reading, keeping fit – keeping alive. And, of course, Mother!

Mother always goes on about Gordon's hair as well as mine, bewailing the disappearance of his babyhood golden curls. Once, when she was moaning about his short cropped hair, I told her that one of his friends had hair exactly like that.
My brother and many of his friends are cyclists, and I think the short hair could be to do with that.

'Oh well, he's copying him then,' was her reply.

There has always been this 'copying' about many things that her children do, so not acknowledging that we are people of any strength or real character of our own. So I know that if I tell her Vanessa likes my hair, and Mother should meet her and find out that she has short layered hair like mine, it will be that I am copying my Minister.

After sticking up the envelope to my daughter with sellotape, I begin my usual routine and get ready for bed, then read for an hour or so marking quotes down on my piece of scrap paper bookmark. I allow myself three squares of chocolate while I am reading, and so the last thing to do is clean my teeth. Tonight I can get no more out of the toothpaste tube, so I cut it open as I always do. That way it will do for at least another week.

Everything runs out, I think, including time, including life, especially Mother's life.

And including time for Christmas shopping, I laugh.

Writing to Imogen has made me think of the children, then the grandchildren, then Christmas presents, and suddenly I know what I will do for Mother.

Beautiful Dreamer

Chapter 29

Well, it is not the gypsy caravan or camper van. It is not going to be around the world, or even just to France, but at least I have got some sort of an outing together for Mother.
We are off to the big Tesco's Supermarket nearby for shopping and coffee. This has taken some weeks to organise because I have had to wait for a Carer to be free to come with us. Sylvia, one of my creative writing students, will be accompanying us too. I pick her up and we collect Mother who was already waiting with her coat and hat on.

Then we have the pantomime of the wheelchair. Mother had a custom-built one provided by the Social Services, because they really need to be made to individual specification according to weight, height and nature of disability. Having got it out to my car, for a moment I am worried that it won't go in until I think of removing the parcel shelf at the back of the car, so opening up the boot. We fold down the chair and take off of the bits that stuck out.

I go back into the Home to get Mother, only to be told that I should not have taken the chair yet because they need it to transport her to the car park. Defeat has begun to settle in when the Manager says we could use one of the communal ones, just for that short distance. Then it is Mother into the car, wheelchair back to base; then on arriving, her own wheelchair out of boot and all unfolded and put together again, and taken around to Mother in the car. Only as we approach the entrance of the store, do I see a large notice, 'Wheelchairs for Customer Use'!

Throughout the short journey from the Home, Mother was beside me in the car and rambled on about this and that, and wasn't this nice, and how she wished she could go for a longer drive, and why wouldn't I take her to France.

'Mother I can't get myself there,' I said between my teeth, stifling a scream. In the back of the car, with Sylvia, was the Carer who has come with us. She was obviously very nervous about cars, and was equally rambling on and on about how Ellie must be quiet because her daughter was driving and must be left to concentrate.

I thought of the many car rides with Mother where I have screamed at her, that if she did not shut up, I would crash the car. In the period before the purchase of my house, Rafe had a girl friend who often came to stay in the house that we all shared with my ex-husband.

'Will you have to get a house big enough to have a room for Rafe's girlfriend?' needled Mother one Sunday.

'No,' I screamed.

She knew how to press the right buttons to infuriate me. did not have to provide a bedroom, but she knew that if made to, I would have. What she was rubbing in was that I let everyone run my life. She had fashioned me to be like that, so I would live her life for her, but still jeers at me for letting others do the same.

'Will you have to have a room for the girl friend?'

'I don't have to do anything!' I slammed my foot on the brake. Fortunately the woman close behind me stopped her car in time, but she drove past me with the two fingered gesture and the mouthing. I didn't blame her. She could have got out and hit me, Mother nearly killed us all.

Anyway, this drive is over and Mother is safely in the chair and we are walking towards the clothes and other goods, on the other side to the food section. The Carer has Mother's wheelchair and I have the trolley. Christmas is not far away, and here I am yet again taking my mother to do her Christmas shopping as I have done since my father died. I start throwing things into the trolley. Bath salts for Valerie, a pretty notebook for Hayley. 'Look,' I say, 'these hankies would do for Gordon. He always likes a hanky.'

'I want to give him a tie.' I turn to the ties and begin twirling round the moving stand.

'Here you are,' I show one to Mother. 'He will like that.'

'No, I want to choose it myself.' So I twirl it around again until she has pointed to the tie she likes. I begin to walk more slowly and take her down all the aisles.

'I want a photo frame,' says Mother. 'I can put my picture of Mum in it.'

There are gift boxes of sweets and biscuits ahead, and we stop by them. This time I stand back while Mother chooses a box of chocolates for Victor and his family.

I have suggested coffee next, so now here we are. While the Carer, Delia, wheels Mother off to the toilet. Sylvia and I choose coffee and buns for all of us and wait. Mother has chosen all the rest of her presents, and the box of Christmas cards. We bought a large jar of sweets for all the Carers – the only way we can repay them. Money for today's help has been refused as it is not permitted.

So here we are. We settle Mother as near to the table as possible, and while they all chat I recall the many outings when Sylvia has helped me with Mother: the teas, the parks, the films and even the visits to Stately Homes. I remember that not having done sufficient homework once, it turned out that the guided tour meant lots of stairs which Mother, then about eighty-four, puffed her way around until Sylvia and I had to put her on a seat somewhere while we finished the tour.

When we took her to see 'Mrs Doubtfire,' it wasn't until we arrived at the cinema that we discovered the film was being shown on the screen which was at the very top of the building. Again, we dragged Mother up stairs with difficulty, fear and guilt. I was so relieved to have my friend with me because we really thought she was going to die!

Another time Sylvia chose 'Sense and Sensibility' for her. We both thought Mother would love the clothes and the old days and the beautiful ladies, but she nagged and muttered throughout the film. I don't know what the complaints were, but a few days later, Sylvia went to see the film again because my mother had totally ruined it for her.

On another Christmas shopping occasion, I had taken Mother first to her favourite lunch place in Hampton Hill, and then had to double back towards Kingston to collect Sylvia.

We then went back to the Hampton Hill area to the supermarket which contained teas and plenty of things suitable for gifts. My friend was kindly coming to help my mother with her Christmas shopping.

'By the time we pick Sylvia up, and get back again, it will be time to go home,' nagged Mother in the car. 'How would you feel if I ordered you to do something?'

Yet more inward screaming! Mother you order me all the time, Sylvia has ordered nothing of me, she is coming to help you, and she does not drive.

My mind is jogged back to the present and our trip today, as Delia is speaking to me.

'Can we get her a little bottle of brandy? She asks nervously. 'She often says she would like a little drink in the evenings, and it does seem to make her sleep better.'

Yes, I think to myself, and then maybe she won't be waking up and falling out of bed by trying to go and telephone her mum. This has happened so many times recently, and in a way I admire her for not pressing the button to call for help. I see that spirit, again, which took her out on her gallivanting and gadding about, in spite of all the back biting.

In Tesco's café, Mother and Sylvia talk about the shops and shopping, and all the places she and Sylvia liked to go to, like Kew gardens and Ealing. Sylvia always travelled further afield than I ever did, even though she does not have a car..

'I wonder if we could get her a cassette player, too,' asks Delia tentatively. 'She won't watch television or listen to the radio that we put on in the lounge, but she does talk about liking music.'

'Can we get her one here?'

'No, but I'll get it for you. There is a place near where I live.'

How kind she is, I think. I know Delia is a Career in the Home half a day, but she also cares for her disabled husband at home.

'I'll try to find some Beatles tapes,' I say. 'I doubt whether I can find, 'One Fine Day,' on its own, and I know she won't want the rest of the opera.'

Later, the reverse trip is done, and we are back at the Home.

'Thank you,' I say to the Manager, 'for releasing Delia.'

It has been a good day, Mother chose a blouse for herself after the tea, and other than the first few presents which I threw into the trolley, she has chosen everything else herself. When I showed Mother's new blouse to one of the Carers, partly for them to mark it as hers, remembering the clothes that went missing at Fawsett House, she tells me they are having a clothes sale next Thursday. Churchfield arrange for a clothes company to come in twice a year because most of the residents can't get out to do any shopping, and don't all have relatives to help with buying clothes. She asks if I can come to help my mother choose things, but I tell her it is my writing class on Thursday.

'Never mind, I'll get Delia to go through her things, and see what she needs.'

'No,' I say, 'let her do it herself. Let her choose her own clothes.'

'We can't spare someone to push her round. Delia can just pop in and out, quickly.'

'What time does it end?' I ask.

'Oh, about twelve thirty, and its starts around eleven.'

My class this week starts at ten and ends at twelve, then we usually have a bring-and-share lunch.

'You can do the class in my house,' says Sylvia. She lives only two minutes from the Home. 'You'll have to skip lunch.'

'I'll be here by ten past twelve,' I say.

As Sylvia and I walk out to the car, I think of my mother choosing the tie. I think of her trying to get out of bed to use the commode without calling for help. I think of the time when she had waited in vain for Gordon to come and put a battery in her radio and told me that she had finally done it herself because she was not going to let it beat her. I wonder at the mixture my mother is, and

I wonder how that spirit might have developed had she not been put in the role of 'Silly Little Nellie,' because that suited everyone.

As I drive home I think of what Delia said when she asked if someone could buy my mother a cassette player. She reminded me that Mother won't watch television, and I suddenly get a brainwave about what to ask Hayley to give her grandmother for Christmas: a video of her favourite film Genevieve. Maybe that would get her to the television, and maybe then she would watch it more often I remember how Mother has always talking about Genevieve and the Yellow Rolls Royce, both about outings or holidays, both films about luxury and posh people – just other forms of the gypsy caravan and the camper van I suppose. We arrive at Sylvia's house and go in for lunch.

'You are so good to help with my mum,' I say to her.

'No,' she says. 'You know, one of my best Christmases was that time we helped your mum to do her shopping in Hampton.'

I think of all the kindness Mother receives, but does not acknowledge, help from Sylvia, from Hayley. Suddenly I remember one of the Sunday outings with Mother, and what Rafe said to me when I got home.

'Have you been out with Nan? he asked.

'Yes, to Richmond Park,' I replied.

'Oh,' he said. 'That's awful. I looked in the paper, at the television programmes, and guess what was on this afternoon? The Yellow Rolls Royce!'

When I told my mother she could not believe that Rafe knew that much about her.

If only she had recognised all that could have been for her, all that was good going on around her.

Chapter 30

I'm having a jewellery party today, and with Christmas presents in mind I was hoping to be lucky and get a good commission on sales. We have all tried on, looked at, admired, and desired the expensive ear-rings and things, have earned some free earrings, and now we are having our bring and share lunch. After my daily meals of soya or plain rice and beans or lentil soup, the quiche and cold chicken are like nectar.

I do keep a bag of cheap chicken portions in the freezer and allow myself one occasionally. My favourite meal is a salmon steak, and when I sometimes treat myself to that, I have only half and save the other half for a few weeks later.

Another variation to my evening choices is that I try to save a few slices of the roast meat when out with Mother Some pubs give you far too much. I wrap it in paper napkins, take in home in my handbag, and it can sometimes do three evening meals.

My lunches are usually one sardine with a small salad, cheap off-cuts of cold meat from my local supermarket, and occasionally my absolute favourite which is cheese on toast. I have that rarely, not just because of cost, but because it is not so healthy as the sardine – just as I reject the more desirable cheap dinner options of fish fingers and fried eggs.

But today I don't have to think of the price of the food on offer, and suspend knowledge of what is healthy and what is not.

Eating straight after the jewellery show, I suddenly remember how my mother so often asked me if she would look smarter if she wore earrings.

'So, it isn't just glamour then? Sylvia asks. ` It is smartness too?` I have told her my theory about jewellery and glamour, and wanting to look like a cherished woman.

I start to wonder, whether 'smart' is any different from 'glamour? I suppose it is in a way.

Mother was always asking me things like that. When I was a teenager she asked me what 'grooming' meant. I did not know myself at that time. Why did she never know these things? Why didn't she try to find out? Was it again to do with the aristocratic blood in her veins? Did she need to have someone to do the grooming for her, as well as dress her? Only now, after a lifetime do I see the light. All she ever wanted was a lady's maid, and tried so hard to make me be that for her.

I explain my theory that jewellery is two things, an expression of worth, and also a sexual allure. Surely, the use of adornments from early history must be that? The glitter of a bracelet leading the man's eyes up the soft downy arm to the face. The sparkling earrings taking his gaze, which then travels along the jaw, down the neck – and to the boobs.
Someone tells me I am 'analysing too much.' How many times has that been said to me? How I long to say, 'but I like analysing.'

The woman who said it is Enid. I have not met her before; a neighbour of Naomi who was brought along to make up the numbers. She is very overweight and tells us that she goes to Weight Watchers.

'What my mother did not understand was that nothing makes you look smart if you have buttons off your coat, or even something spilled down your front. Not to mention grubby finger nails.'

'Did she try nail polish? Mavis asks, she is Sylvia's sister in- law. 'Some people think that makes you look smarter, and it sometimes makes you look after your nails better.'

'Oh yes, she did wear nail varnish, sometimes, but with the dirty finger nails underneath.'

'How was your mother last time you saw her? Hilary asks.

'Still wanting to go home to her mother,' I say. 'She`s wanting me to get a Spiritual Healer in. She thinks they might help her to get home.'

'Is she religious? Mavis asks, 'I mean – going to a Spiritualist Church.'

'No not really.' I think for a minute. 'No, she went for the healing hands all over her and messages from the other side telling her what she wanted to hear.'

'A load of mumbo jumbo, if you ask me,' said Enid.

'Well people have always gone in for that. My mother used to go to fortune tellers, whenever she got the chance,' I tell them.

'Fortune tellers and horoscopes, says Naomi. 'And now it's Spiritual Healers.'

'There are spiritual healers and spiritual healers,' I say.

'What do you mean,' asks Mavis.

'Well, the sort that are in my mother's Spiritualist Church, and the new sort I have been to. They don't give you messages. They make you look inside yourself. Get in touch with your spiritual self.'

'I'm only just beginning to understand,' says Naomi, 'that book you let me borrow.'

'It's the new age spirituality' I say, bringing in the puddings.
'Books, groups, counsellors, it's all about looking inwards now, examining your motives, changing life patterns, moving on. Yes, looking how to move on instead of...I don't know, instead of being told everything will be all right.'

'Like your Mum's been told?'

`And nothing is ever right ?` Sylvia said.

'I understand the new idea is all to do with healing and
believing,' I say.

'Too late for your mum now,' says Enid.

'Nothing's ever too late,' I reply, giving her an extra-large slice of cheese cake and sniggering at the way she tucks into it. I think, she's not going to move on, Weight Watchers or no Weight Watchers.

'Haven't the psychologists told you that your mother won't change now?' Sylvia asks, more gently.

'Yes, but I won't accept it. Why else is she still alive?'

'Do you mean it's not too late for her to get better, or that it is too late for her to have the things she wants? Hilary asks. 'Both.' I say. 'Who would like more wine?

'What hasn't she got?' Enid asks. 'I work in a Home. Did Naomi tell you? I think that my clients have nothing to complain of. They are all clean and fed.'

'Oh I forgot,' Naomi looks embarrassed. 'Enid is a Carer in a Home near Richmond.

'So what hasn't your mum got?' Enid asks again.

'Travel,' I say. 'Oh, and sex.' I laugh.

'Oh she's had sex,' says Mavis. 'She had you at least, and haven't you got brothers? A sister?'

'You can have babies without having much of a sex life,' I say.

'I can't bear to think of old people that way at all,' says Sylvia.

'They all need it. We all need it forever,' I say, for I am sure of this.

'Oh, it's disgusting,' says Enid. 'We've got this Nun in the Home, she lies on her bed half the day masturbating. Every time you go into her room, there she is, with her drawers off and her legs wide open and her hand…. Well, you know.

I think to myself, if you've done without an orgasm all your life, then you might as well give up now.'

'That is exactly what you are not going to do,' I say. 'Give up, I mean at a deep level, in terms of the misery that the lack brings you. Even if you don't know what it is you want. Or you do, like Mum.'

'There is an old man in the same Home where my dad is,' says Mavis. 'They catch him tossing himself off all the time.'

'Disgusting,' continues Enid.

'Pity the nun and the old man can't get together,' laughs Naomi.

'What I say,' Mavis says, 'is what you've never had you never miss.'

'Do you think if you lived all your life on an island – I don't know – a lone couple shipwrecked, you were born there, orphaned – and you had a brain the size of a planet, you would not feel some enormous inner something? Some mental thirst?'

I am seething inside, but I can never show it. I remember the days when my children were young, when all I had was domesticity, thinking to myself that there was something I wanted but didn't know what it was.

'Sex seems to me to be like money. The people who have it always tell people who don't that it doesn't make any difference.' I turn to Enid. 'Do you like your job?

'Course not,' says Enid, giving me a look. 'But I believe in earning my living.'

Pity you don't earn enough to buy some jewellery, I think, as she is the only one who has not placed an order. I might have got better earrings.

'It's all wiping old ladies bums, isn't it?' Enid says. 'Of course I don't like it. Who would!' Enid stomps out to the bathroom.

She has touched a raw spot. Working in a Care Home is the one job I know I could get. I can't face doing it because I feel that would be yet another example of the rough end of woman hood, when I have had hardly any of the other side.

Besides, I would not earn much, probably not much more than I receive in benefits, and I would be too outraged by the injustices which have put me there. This country owes me the result of two inequitably run divorces.

'I'm sorry,' says Naomi. 'I didn't know what she was like. don't know her very well.'

'I certainly wouldn't like to be a resident in her Home,' says Hilary. 'Where my old aunt was, the Carers loved the people. They said you had to clean them up in a way that made them feel okay about it,'

'Anyway,' said Enid coming back into the room. 'They are nasty, those old people. They bite and scratch you. You have to fight to get their medicine down them. What I say is, this, if they don't want their medicine, they don't want to live.
Why should we have to work so hard to get them to eat or get them to take their pills, if they don't want to?'

'There may be more behind all that than the obvious,' I say in defence. 'It may not be a way of saying they don't want to live.'

'What then?' Enid snaps at me.

'I haven't worked it out yet,' I say thoughtfully. 'I'm trying to understand by studying my mother, and the other people in her Home.'

After they have nearly all gone, it is only Naomi and me, and while she is doing the washing up, I think again of my mother wanting to look smart by wearing earrings and I remember the one time Mother did try an Adult Education class, a self-improvement one too, you could say. She has always wished that she had what she called 'a better speaking voice.' She would have liked elocution lessons, and in the Adult Education brochure that I showed her she spotted a class on 'Public Speaking.' I tried to explain that I didn't think it was quite what she wanted, but she insisted on going.

When I saw her the day after the first class, she was almost shaking, and there was certainly a sense of panic about her.

The term's course had begun with a general talk on self-presentation, including appearance, and began at the beginning with the most basic aspect of that – personal freshness. I knew before she explained, just why Mother was telling me she was never going again, but she was kidding herself it was something else.

'They were all arriving in cars,' she spoke in a rush. 'Everyone had a car or had someone meeting them in a car. I was the only one walking on my own.' She threw an accusing look in my direction.

'They were all being picked up. They were all coming up in cars.' She kept repeating theses sentences. This would certainly have been a humiliation for her, I knew, this desire to be seen to be loved. But, deep down, I knew what had caused the panic. It was the personal freshness bit.

My mother always had a smell about her. From the age of about forty, until she went into a Home and was regularly washed, there was always that distinct odour. It was mostly due to underwear worn too long and then, later, unchecked urine incontinence, and maybe at times a vaginal discharge as well. Certainly, from her mid-forties I could remember the whiff always being there. She left damp patches on chairs too, and could be seen scrabbling for newspapers or anything nearby, like an old cardigan, to push under herself. If the class teacher talked of being sure of personal freshness then she would have believed that everyone was looking at her. She would have felt humiliated.

'Did she ever do anything about it? Naomi asks when I tell her about it.

'Well yes, she did. She put things under herself. But my first husband was always washing the chairs after she had visited us.'

'Did she ever go to see a doctor?'

'Yes,' I say, 'and she got them to give her a biopsy once. She believed it was something seriously wrong, something to do with her womb, I suppose, although she had never talked of the problem to me.'

'You've said she did not change her underwear every day, but couldn't she have used pads? Talked to a girl friend or something? Done something, instead of all those years of worrying and feeling ashamed?'

'She didn't have girl friends,' I say. 'She didn't talk of anything really. All she ever talked about was of wanting to go abroad, or moving house. I am not sure if she really understood anything about the world around her. That generation always called urine `water`, and if one of us wet the bed when we were small, she just hung the sheet out to dry, so I guess she thought that she only had to dry her knickers.'

Naomi and I drain the last bottle of wine. Thinking of the earrings and wanting to be smart, and saying to me she did not know how to 'go about`' getting herself abroad reminds me that she did not know how to cope. She certainly did not know how to manage her own body. Again I think of her claims to nobility and how she may not have it in her blood to deal with these things.

'Sorry about Enid,' says Naomi again. 'I am glad that she could not wait for me. She had to be at the Home by two.'

I think about what Enid said about biting and scratching and remember my mother scratching Valerie's face, like some animal. I tell Naomi of my theory about sexual jealousy.

'It certainly figures,' says Naomi, 'all the Carers are a lot younger than their clients.'

'Yes, the old people would assume they are all sexually active, or at least that they still have hope in that side of life. They would see the Carers as having time on their side.'

Naomi is quiet as she puts her coat on. 'You know your mother's reaction to that class – panic, even shaking I think you said? Actually, I think she was frightened.'

'Of what? I ask.
'Well, she was frightened that her smell had been noticed, might even have been commented upon.'

*

Frightened?

Mother has always looked frightened, I think, as I wave Naomi away. Sometimes she has that arrogant, stubborn look, but at other times she looks pleading, and yes, scared.

Running scared, that is what she was like in the last year leading up to the collapse which put her into a Home.

Now, having tidied my house after the jewellery party, I sit and enjoy my room for a while, feeling my friends and their chatter all round me. Then I go to my bed to finish a book and write up my quotes, before settling down to write to Imogen. I tell my daughter about the party and my new earrings, and a bit about how her grandmother is getting on. Then I find myself biting my pen and remembering that last year, before Mother's near death experience, alone down by her beloved river.

In a way, I suppose it all began one evening when she telephoned me six times. I had taken her out for most of that Sunday, and I was trying to catch up on my exercises, putting my washing away, and planning to read before the routine of yoga and meditation. Mother had telephoned to say thank you for the day and then asked if she could live with me. This went on all evening and I felt the old panic of being taken over by her, of not being able to get on with life, not being about to say 'no.'

After the sixth call I told her that tomorrow I would change my telephone number, which I did, but it took until Wednesday to take effect, so I still got the calls.

On the last day she said, almost sounding gleeful, 'oh you're changing your number tomorrow, aren't you?

It was as though it were a game to her. She did not think for one moment that I would keep it up, I suppose it was a bit of a lover's tiff to her. Valerie told me later that Mother had said to her that she had 'fallen out' with me.

The need for a lover too, I think, as I prepare to bath and begin my meditation programme. One of my friends who had an argument with a very clingy and demanding friend once told me how, every time the friend banged the phone down on her, she felt that the other girl was behaving as she would to a lover, that she was getting some kind of thrill out of it all – out of the argument that led to the banging down of the phone.

Mother treating me as a lover, I realise, as I begin my yoga session. Well, she thinks I am everything else, and what about the time she accused me of wanting her to marry so that I did not have to 'do it' – be her husband?

I want a lover more than I want anything else at the moment, but like Bernard, I face my aloneness, admit it to myself. But for some, like mother, they take any deep misery out on someone else. It comes out in some way, destructive to themselves or to others.

Years ago, I said to Gordon that I believed our mother would not be alive if it were not for the adrenaline, the energy, she got from riling me. 'I know,' he said. 'She winds you up.
I've watched her doing it. She doesn't do it to me.' Well… she has well-schooled me to being a victim, and she would not do it to him. Although she did not like men, she adored her sons.

I fill the bath and start my short yoga routine, thinking of the buzz and excitement of having someone else to fight with, someone on whom to bang down the phone. What else was all this now to her, but a lover's tiff?

Obviously I still saw her after that episode, and I still phoned her, but I never relented on the telephone number. She had lost her lifeline. During this period, telephones calls came from hospitals, because Mother would telephone for ambulances frequently. She would be taken into hospital, discharged, and then she would telephone for an ambulance again and be taken back to hospital. She called doctors at all times of the day and night.

I went to her doctor as, somehow, Mother had got through to him on his private line. He had no idea how she had managed that, and he described his treatment by her as being 'abusive.' I wondered again at her seemingly inadequacy on so many levels and yet she could be so cunning when she needed it. How did she know how to get hold of the doctor's private number? She telephoned all sorts of local council departments and got through, even where most human beings these days can hardly get through to anybody.

'What does she want from you?' I asked the doctor.

'She wants me to tell her that everything is all right,' he replied.

Tell her she will never die, I think.

Mother telephoned doctors, ambulances, Social Workers, and even the police. She was in and out of hospital and we were all being called to them. We visited back and fore.

Twice she was put into a local hospital for the mentally challenged. We visited and felt sick as we left our mother standing looking at us through the glass of a locked door. Then we had the final telephone call when she had collapsed out of doors, and somebody else had called an ambulance.

Lying in my bubbles I think of the Kingston's Carer's Association, which looks after people caring for the elderly and the disabled. None of the people really understood my mother, and talked of her 'anxiety.' What I had seen in that last year before she went onto Residential Care – the telephoning doctors and the police – was terror: the fear of being alone, of illness, of eventual death. Maybe it was the terror of dying alone that was the worst.

I have always seen the going out – the extreme of going out which meant ignoring basic care of home or self or children – as running away, and perhaps it was always a running away from fear. But whatever the demon was from which she ran all my life, I am not sure. Maybe it was one of the effects of having been sexually abused.

I suppose I see all kinds of behaviour as a running – escape and an expression of fear. I see it in friends who are more often out than in. I see it in all of us who like to escape by drinking and smoking. The fact of mortality is one of the greatest goblins from which we all hide, often as much through material possessions or prestige, as in drinking and smoking or going out. Someone even said that dieting, exercise, even colouring our hair, are all to do with not facing age and ultimate death.

But there are other horrors to run from, like parental rejection or abuse, or some long buried hurt, and there are still yet more ways of hiding from them. I know friends who have unbearable realities. They cope by non-stop talking, fast and loud. You can see people looking at them in public places, and I know they have prevented others hearing themselves speak. It rises to a screeching and squawking, and it seems to me that they are silencing the goblins inside their heads, who want their attention.

To scream can be to silence the truth. I know that if two police officers stood at my front door, and I just knew that they were about to give me news of the death of one of my children, I would scream and scream, not because of the news, but to prevent it being given to me. Is this why some of the Home residents walk up and down? Why some of them babble and babble at you, with words which do not make sense?

My poor lonely frightened Mother. Just before she went into the Home, I bumped into a friend I had not seen for ages, but who knew my mother. 'You know,' she said, as we shared news in the shops. 'I saw your mother recently, sitting on a seat in Surbiton, really early in the day, I was driving friends who had been staying with me to the Station, and there she was. At eight in the morning.

I can only surmise that Mother woke up at the crack of dawn, after a time could not bear lying there any longer, threw clothes on, made a quick cup of tea and went out.
There would have been plenty of buses at that time of day, but there would have been no shops or cafés open. She could not stand to be on her own in that flat, in her head. But was it just loneliness, or was it also fear?

Allowing the towel to be my cuddles, I settle down to my meditation. Afterwards, I slip the towel off and look at my body in my full length mirror, and remember what finally put my mother in a Home. What actually happened was never told clearly to me.
After the near death at the riverside, and subsequent hospital stay, she did actually go home for a few days. She was not coping well, the Social Worker later told us, but I do not know in what way. Victor visited the flat the first weekend, and it was a neighbour who gave him the news that she had been taken into hospital from where she was quickly put into the Residential Home. The neighbour told my brother that there were rumours she had been trying to leave the flat– and she was undressed, possibly naked.

As I return my body to its loneliness under pyjamas and dressing gown, what suddenly comes back to me is the one time Mother and I stayed in Worthing overnight, so that I could give her a longer weekend. We shared a room in the hotel, and I dressed and undressed myself inside the shower cubicle. When I came out of the en-suite shower, I found Mother sitting on the bed completely naked. And I knew it was because she desired her body to be seen.

I go downstairs to make a light supper which is all I need after all the lovely lunch food brought my friends. I am playing with the idea that the fear seen in my mother is not just a fear of dying, but also of dying without having experienced sexual fulfilment, without having had the affairs with soldiers which would have been `something to remember.'

Later the following morning, I receive another call from the Home. Mother has had yet another fall. Once again it happened when she was trying to get to the telephone. I rush to the Home.

'Who were you trying to phone? I ask when I arrive at her bed.
'Mum.'

'What number where you going to ring?' I enquire.

'5321'

My old number! The one I had before I changed it, and she still remembers.

'So she must think you are Mum,' says Anna, 'if she is ringing her 'mum' on your number.' She and Hayley have both come with me, and all their children. The children stare at their grandmother. She is dribbling as she often does these days and I cannot stand it. The saliva runs from her mouth and settles in slime which hangs from her neck know I am disgracefully squeamish, but I have called a Carer who now comes and wipes Mother with kitchen roll. I keep some handy, though I know I won't be able to bring myself to use it.

Tea, squash and biscuits are brought to us. It is something to do. Mother does not talk to the little children, but just keeps repeating that she wants to go home, and that she wants a jacket like the one Anna is wearing. The conversations have always been the same, she wants to move, she wants to go on holiday, she still wants to go to France, but most of all now she wants to go home to Mum and the shop.

The 'playing card lady' bears down on us, and Freddie is scared, as am I. It is time to go, but as we all stand up and say goodbye,

little Freddie walks closer to my mother and says, 'I want a hug.' I am filled with wonder and gratitude.
Mother gives him a small hug, but does not look any less unhappy. I feel sad; everything is too late now, nothing will ever make any difference.

The two girls come into my house and we talk while the children find things to do in my toy box.

Now I am finally on my own, and I think it was good of Anna to come in view of the history with my mother. When the divorce between me and her father was announced, my mother used to get the thirteen-year-old on her own and tell her it was all her father's fault. For many years, right into the days when Anna was in sixth form college, Mother would arrange to meet her for coffee then, when she got her there, would go on and on, saying that the divorce was caused by the children's father joining a sailing club.

Those coffee sessions always remind me of the times I met her when the two older girls were tiny and, pinned by the offer of tea and something to eat, I had to sit in silence while she went on and on at me saying that I was an uncared for poor housewife. A failed woman.

All the help I have had with Mother! All the places and people I have approached for nearly thirty years – a church minister, counsellors, Social Workers, doctors, psychologists, the head of the Carer's organisation. The last thing the head man of that organisation ever said to me was 'change your telephone number.'

I did, and what did she do? She went and telephoned Anna instead, sometimes as many as thirteen times in a day. Once at seven o'clock on a Saturday morning when, as well as having two children, my daughter was a teacher during the week and wanted a lie in. She never gave up, until she went into Residential Care, trying to wear my daughter down into giving her my new phone number.

My Christmas cards are posted, and now, after the girls and their families have gone, I sort through my pile of presents and re-assess what is still to be bought. For the first time in thirty years, there is less to do for Mother. We brought the presents in

Tesco's and the few cards she wanted to send have all been done. Of course she wants to send a card to her mum.

The Carers have said they will wrap her presents, or they will get her to do it with them as an `activity`. Only a few years ago, when I was doing all her wrapping for her, she said to me, 'you make yourself do it, don't you? I suppose I am a lazy person really.' Handy! And I think, not for the first time that, at the age I am now, she was being waited on by me.
No, younger. In the days when I was running after her and she was 'enjoying herself', she was in her early to mid-fifties.
Would she have looked after her own mother if alive, instead of being out and about on buses?

But I also remember a time when I did not get round to the flat to wrap the last present, and she brought it on Christmas Day. She clearly had not been able to find ribbon or string, and had tied the holly paper up by sewing it with needle and thread. Was this just the old inadequacy, the laziness, or the aristocratic genes? My kind Rafe, a little boy at the time, said he felt `sorry for 'Nan.' If she really had no sellotape, maybe what she did could be said to be resourceful. Somebody I told thought so. So is it all a question of interpretation?

Remembering the sewn present brings to mind one of the rare occasions when Mother invited me round to tea with my children. She had bought a plain sponge cake, and had clearly realised it needed decoration. She had not remembered to buy cherries or dolly mixtures or proper icing, but had sprinkled the top of the cake with granulated sugar. I thought she could have done better. But I suppose she did do something, she did try and have a go? Rafe again felt sorry for her.

It was a Christmas episode which was a precursor to the, 'can I come and live with you' telephone call that made me change my telephone number. It was another instance of non-stop calls, and maybe without it I would not have reacted so strongly the next time.

Gordon and I had decided to buy Mother clothes as her present, and Hayley offered to buy her a winter coat. I went shopping for a skirt and jumper, while Hayley bought the coat on her own. I took these gifts on Christmas Eve, because she was spending

Christmas day with Victor as usual – as her failing major carer of a daughter had fobbed off her duty to her brother.

A few days after Christmas, the calls started to come. She did not like any of the clothes. You should never buy clothes as a present without the person there to try them on. I received nine of these calls in one evening.

Well, in a way she was right. She buys so few clothes herself that it would have been nice for her to have chosen her own, but any shopping with Mother is hard work. I took all the clothes back and gave her the money. The clothes were actually from Hayley and Gordon – but it was I who got the nine calls and had to return the clothes.

I think the reason that I rejected the idea of taking Mother shopping was because of an earlier incident concerning a wedding ring. Mother's original one had long ago worn very thin and finally broken. For years she had been buying a series of cheap rings from Kingston market to wear on that finger. At last, the Christmas before the clothes episode, Hayley gave her a proper wedding ring. However it did not fit, but who had to go with Mother to change it?

To take Mother anywhere meant picking her up, dropping her near the shops or café, going off to park then walking back to the glowering look for having been so long. In the case of the ring it meant that, once I had done the parking bit, I had to take her for coffee, half carrying her, or so it seemed. Then the long walk to the jeweller's, supervising the trying on, then lunch and the journey in reverse, and all to be told, when we got back to her flat, that I was unkind not to stay for tea.

At least there was one of the lighter moments, though, on that trip. Mother pointed out what neither Hayley nor I had thought of. As she looked at the shiny new wedding ring, Mother remarked that people would think that she had just got married!

Christmas memories abound as another Christmas approaches, memories too of laziness and resourcefulness.
Interesting that her use of me could be caused by inadequacy but called for certain skills in manipulation. Memories of persecution and memories of fear, and now she has yet another fall.

Chapter 31

Mother has had another fall, and this time she fell on to her face. I was told that her face was bruised, but also she had fallen in such a way that they suspected she may have suffered a mini stroke. Mother has spent the last two days in hospital under observation, which had me jumping every time the telephone rang, expecting the worst news.

This morning I heard from Churchfield House that she is to go back there today, and the thought of her, of her bleak life stretching ahead, brings fresh hope that she still might watch the new videos she had for Christmas. Hayley did manage to get Mother's two favourite films for her, but so far she has not wanted to look at them.

Thinking of Christmas brings back the memory where she said she was lazy about wrapping presents. What is lazy?
What does the word mean? There are many things I do happily and well, some I do with exhaustion and resentment, and others I refuse to do at all. I know that this last comes from anger at having to do anything I really don't like when I have so little in my life that I really do like. Or what I would really like is not available to me.

Does any mother ever have a chance to be lazy? Just the mere fact of having children to look after, sufficiently well to prevent them being put into care, involves a lot more effort than just not being lazy. The degree of our mother's neglect is a testament surely to being overworked, worried, fed up, at least, and almost certainly immeasurably depressed.

We children certainly went to school the worst dressed in our classes. My sister and I both had our hair combed out by teachers in front of our classes. There was no money for clothes, and in her early housework years Mother had not only no washing machine, but also no hot water. Other mothers did it all with similar conditions, but with what other advantages? Extended family help? A happy marriage? A happy bed to look forward to?

Our mother could not sleep when we were young. She would lie awake, then take sleeping pills with the result that she found it hard to get out of bed in the morning, never mind get us ready, or take us to school.

Consider what her life was like in those days. Dad was away in the shop, not coming home at all during the working week, so what did she have to look forward to as she went to bed in the evenings? What was there to look forward to each day? Mother had little social life, no sympathy, no comfort, no love, no man or sex she could warm to. Nothing to balance the drudgery.

To achieve a fulfilling sex life seems to be more difficult for women than men. This is on my mind today and I am disturbed. Thinking of my mother's lonely days in her thirties adds to the angry feelings I have had since reading a news item earlier today. A woman who went to a Dating Agency has been murdered by a man she met through it. I met my last husband that way, and have been considering trying that route again. The woman was young and a doctor. Why did someone like that have to resort to such means to get her needs met? Why do I?

As I dress and make up my face, I decided I am going to write an article. I have thought it out and will call it, 'Married, Dead or Deviant,' for it seems to me that all men of my age are one of those at least. I shall address the fact that men seek younger women, and so as time goes by, our chances of meeting a partner decreases. The deviant ones may want us because the young girl would not put up with them.

My friends have told me not to try again. 'How could you after you last experience?' They say. They do not know that I have been trying for many years, answering advertisements from Lonely Hearts columns in newspapers. I study the form sent by the Agency I have chosen now, and laugh at the section for interests.

For all the men I have recently met on the telephone have assured me that they have the same interests as me, like the same music, are passionate about learning. But when I met them, it was clear that they were all thinking, here is a woman who is free, and whose telephone number I have. A handy lay for occasions when I am desperate. I decide to write the article first, before filling in the forms.

*

Afternoon, and here we are again back at the Churchfield House, going through the same routine.

'I want my compact,' Mother demands as I approach. She is back from the hospital and I am staring at the all-blue face.
She is not complaining about that. She is still asking to be taken home.

I wonder if I am getting it all wrong, projecting my feelings on to my mother and assuming that all women need to be fulfilled in every way, which includes experiencing their womanhood to the full.

But what about the compact? Having fallen heavily on her face and finding herself on a stretcher and hearing the Carers clucking over her poor face, what did she do? Cry at having fallen? Cry about the pain? Moan about having to go into hospital? No, she thought of how her face might look and asked the Carers for her compact. To try and cover the damaged face. I look across at her as she tears open the little packet of chocolate buttons I have brought her. There are already little tufts of hair growing on her chin. How long is it since she asked me to bring her lady who used to wax her face?

I was unable to do that, so she has been getting the Carers to shave her. One day a few weeks ago she told me that the male Carer does it now, and I wondered at the humiliation of letting a man shave your face. Is that the final giving up? The end of all sexual hope?

Of course, Mother's personal sexuality has been a mystery to me for a long time. Years ago she went on holiday. I think it was something like a Retreat, certainly some kind of church based respite holiday, in a large country house. Afterwards she told me and my teenage daughters that she was brought tea in bed by a young man and, as we giggled about how lucky she was, she said she would rather have had a nice young girl to bring it to her! Was that because of a preference for girls, or just an abhorrence of men, because of what they had been in her life?

In her first Residential Home, she expressed a round 'O' mouth shock and horror as she told me she had been stripped and washed all over by two male Carers. Maybe many of us would react in the same way because of our own modesty and because we are mostly used to female nurses.

Could it also have been shock at the intimacy with men, who are not the desired sex? How much she has been put off men, sex, and marriage by her own experience of childbirth, housework and abuse, I am not sure. I still believe that I have seen a spark of sexual interest in her. Of course the touching of herself all over could be heterosexual, or not. And of course there were the references to the old women on the buses and the soldiers.

I look at her bruised face and remember the bashed back as she dips into the bag of buttons. Has her body had no greater joy than that of eating, of sitting by the river and having a cake in a café? Days are running out for Mother, and I am breathless. I am gasping to keep hold of the hope that I will get her abroad, the hope that a man will come into the Home and love her, maybe even make love to her.

'Oh have you heard?' Laughs the Carer when I go to be let out of Churchfield later, 'in our sister Home across the river, an old couple of ninety are getting married.'

Floating on air I walk to my car, and nurture all my dreams as I drive home.

Chapter 32

I am back home from Churchfield House and my mind is thinking of Mother's poor face and how her first thought on falling was how it would make her look. Her first request was for her face powder compact.

I am reminded of a poem by Paul Hyland describing a very old lady doing her hair. It is white and it reaches to her waist, so she can braid it and pile it high on top of her head. The lady combs and caresses her hair, and the poet remarks on the miracle of so much hair, that the frail skull can still hold it and it can still find root. For both skull and skin are `pared to a bare necessity.` The hair is her 'glory` and 'its business is to persist.' He calls his poem 'Proper Vanity.' I loved this poem long before I began trying to understand my mother and her sexuality, that journey inspired by a nurse all that time ago.

The poem tells of a woman holding onto the last vestige of her femininity and sensuality, and when I first read it I thought how our gender is fundamental to our identity. The first thing that is said when a baby is born is that it is a girl or a boy.

All the female residents of the Home today were sitting with fluffed hair, for today the hairdresser visited. How much of their misery, depression, dementia is caused by the end of being a sexual woman, so losing identity, so losing oneself? Do we hang on to something, anything, be it the brooch or the glorious hair – or the compact powdered face?

When I came downstairs this morning, before going to visit Mother there was a wedge of things through my letter box, bills and 'bumf' as well as the local paper. Now back home I have a chance to go through it, and find one envelope is neither bill nor junk, but a reply from my Introduction Agency, but I soon bin the details sent to me. A business man interested in bridge and country walks is hardly going to get on with a slightly communist, somewhat philosophic, agoraphobic, Gilbert and Sullivan fan is he?

Now, I flick through the Kingston upon Thames local paper, and read that, in another Home in my borough, two elderly men have fought over a woman resident, and one of them has since died.

So sex is only for the young and beautiful I laughingly question, remembering some of my friend's remarks about feeling sick at the thought of the really elderly `at it.`

I don't know whether to laugh or cry. Should I cry because one caused the death of another, or laugh that desire can last right into the nineties?

*

The following day I am off to Churchfield House again, so soon because of the fall and the bruised face. At last I have remembered to bring out to the car my tape of the Gondoliers, given to me by Anna and her family at Christmas. Mother is still apparently refusing to watch her favourite films on video.

As I drive along enjoying my music, yet another old picture of my mother slides onto my internal screen. I can remember her at a performance of this very opera that I am listening to, on one of the few times I took her with me.

First she scrabbled about at the bottom of her bag, and brought out some old jelly babies, covered with dust and which she kept eating throughout the show. I felt guilty. It was obvious that someone of her generation would have expected to have been taken to the theatre 'proper,' and presented in the foyer with a box of chocolates. Well, there was no foyer, no kiosk to buy boxes of chocolates, as this was an amateur operatic company in a small hall used for various functions. I was a 'poor wife' and the only refreshments available in the interval were tea and biscuits. No chocolates for Mother, not like Dad's lady friend at the Yeoman of the Guard performance.

At the end of the Gondoliers, the identity of the King of Barataria is revealed. He mounts his throne, and his queen mounts and receives a crown too. As the orchestra and chorus sang in adulation and the girl, now queen, was raised on high with the crown upon her head, Mother looked sideways, then down, covering her face, touching her hair.

She looked so wretched and accepting. It was as though she were thinking, 'I will never be a queen; will never be made a fuss of, not like that.' To be queen, is that what she really wants? Is that what we all want?

To be a queen, just sometimes? A queen for a day, by being a bride? To be a queen as a little girl by being chosen to be the fairy doll for the top of the tree? To be loved and cherished, to wear the brooches and the pearls, to be given the box of chocolates, to be seen to be cherished, loved, feel important. Perhaps even to be seen to be ravished, to be someone's darling, and therefore a queen among women.

Wanting the box of chocolates reminds me of when Mother spent an evening with my husband and me, in my 'poor wife' days. She would sit and fidget for a while as we watched television and then say, 'do you ever feel like going out for a little drink?' I felt what she really meant was, don't you have any drink in the house? I would expect as your mother to be properly wined and dined when I visit you.` In those days, we could hardly afford to feed the extra mouth. Indeed, we could hardly feed ourselves.

Often Mother would turn up uninvited to stay. She would knock on my door carrying a small suitcase and say she had had a row with Dad and had come to stay. Shades of packing up her things and getting on the tram to stay with Auntie Nellie?

So here we are again, having tea in the Home. What else is there to do? On the weekly Sunday outings, Mother sometimes spotted me reading something under the table as we sat at elevenses, lunch and tea, and say that I must be very bored. The truth was that a whole day was a lot of time for me to give up, and I usually took mail to catch up on, or even forms to fill in, often forms related to services for Mother.

Whether it was the children, my degree, or something else receiving my attention, she would always say that all she wanted was for me to give her some of my time, so that we could have a quiet talk. What did we ever talk about? 'I can't help it if I am boring,' she would say. 'I don't have much in my life to talk about.' Well get something in your life then. Join a club, or a class. I thought but, did not say.

The only talking we ever did was about the lack of seats, or buses, and we usually went down the well-worn route of her not liking the miserable old bitches at the Day Centre, or not being able to get to this place or that, or anyway friends are not the same as `someone of your own.`

Today I get a brief respite when Mother is taken to the loo, and I notice that her pace is almost at a standstill. I look around. Poor old men and women, is there anybody here that anyone would fancy? I did, once, see a man on television who was ninety-four, and not only was he attractive, but fanciable too. Could a woman of that age ever be that? For that bloom akin to youth's first flush would you need super health, or some inner self worth?

I think about the Dating Agency murder, strip clubs, curb crawlers and call girls. The whole sexual scene seems based on the gratification of men and their needs, and those needs being for youth and beauty. And sometimes, for a young child.

Mother is back in front of me now, and I look at her poor face where the bruises are blue or turning yellow. 'I was hurt,' she says, and I look into her face.

Yes, I think to myself, you have indeed been hurt.

*

I remember a time when I sat with a new man, from an Agency, in a beautiful café, in a beautiful setting, and what went through my mind was that my mother had never had an experience like this. Whenever I have or do anything my mother has not experienced, I feel guilty. Every time she told me she had been ill, and how awful it is to be ill and to live on your own, with no one to bring you a cup of tea, I felt guilty too. The cup of tea again. I feel a heavy weight of responsibility and failure setting upon me.

When I was sitting in my house only a street away from her flat, and she called me to say that she was frightened of the thunderstorm or the fireworks, it was the same. I always felt bad that I was not curing all her ills. Only now do I think that I am not the only person in her world, but I am the only person she ever told. I feel bad now, as I hear daily reports from the Home of Mother's increasing illness and falls. She has cellulites in her legs, a urine infection, and is having blood tests.

But sometimes I wonder if this guilt I feel is really masking my own anger at being singled out as the major carer. Worse, am I angry with myself for not resisting? I have always felt that I am failing her if I am not doing everything that Mother requires of me, to have lived with her, taken her the tea to bed, to have gone round and held her hand during the fireworks or thunderstorm. How she twisted the knife in me in those instances, telling me how it reminded her of the war and the bombing. I feel I should be in the Home with her day and night. I know that a bed would be provided.

'If Mum dies it will be your fault.' Maybe I don't do all she wants because I know it would be useless. A friend once said to me that, if I spent the rest of my life sitting at my mother's feet saying how much I really loved her, she would probably tell me I was talking too much.

*

` 'What's the matter, what's the matter?' ` rasped my mother one day, flinging back at me the words I had just spoken. How many people get that asked of them? There was her chance, her golden opportunity. Gordon was driving her out to the countryside. I was going along to help out, and she had been going on about something and nothing, so I asked her the million dollar question: `What's the matter?` Did I get any thanks for my concern, or some clue at last which might help me to help her? No. Just threw my question back at me tauntingly, as though it were of no use to her at all.

Once I left her sitting in a café while I went off to the loo. When I came back, she told me that the woman at the next table had been speaking to her. She had obviously been listening to my mother and me, and said to Mother how lucky she was to have someone with her who was so kind, so interested, so understanding, so trying to be helpful. Mother looked puzzled as she told me that the woman thought she was lucky to have a daughter like me. .

'What's the matter?` I had asked, and it just bounced off her and come back to me. There have been so many offers of help, so many missed chances.

But I have done that too, missed opportunities in life. In the middle of the last divorce, when I was 'ping-ponging' from one solicitor to another, because no one seemed to have my interests at heart, somebody gave me a piece of paper with the name and number of a solicitor on it. The woman who gave it to me was involved in women's issues, worked for a women's organisation, and that lawyer would possibly have been my salvation. Yet I never pursued it. Was it hopelessness or was it that I even sabotage myself, so that I keep myself in the role I have been trained for?

One of my many forays into the world of healing, a year of two later, took me to a talk by spiritual healers. They stopped in the middle of their show and looked towards me in the middle of all the audience, saying they were aware of an enormous black trauma sitting there. When asked, I spoke about my mother, but did not talk of the abusive marriage and divorce, did not talk of my father's abuse, did not talk of my lifelong exhausted crawl to fulfilment in every area of my life.

I think I must have been dismissive, perhaps led them to believe they had got it wrong. The lady protesting, or just that self-sabotage I have noted in myself from time to time. How I wish I had gone to see them privately. They picked up what nobody else has. I wonder if I carry some enormous trauma from another life, or some black horror passed down in my cell memory from my ancestors. Instead of relief and hope I felt embarrassment and, yes, a wanting to hide from something.

Why do we miss our chances, let a golden moment go by?

In my teenage years, Mother told me that she had just walked into the local child and baby clinic and simply cried and cried, so they gave her a cup of tea. Neither she nor the staff at the clinic probed the crying. The tea, being offered, sympathy, those would have brought Mother such immeasurable – though temporal – balm that for a moment wiped away all her tears, but the main reason for her tears was still there.

So is there nothing that can be done for Mother? I feel exhausted as I drive to the Home. She does not listen to the Beatles music we got her and, so far, she has not watched the video of the Yellow Rolls Royce. Is there anything that can be done for me? Still no details have come in the post of the man I would like to meet, and I am sitting opposite Mother as she moans that she would like to go home, that her mum needs her, and that she wants to go abroad.

'But you won't go on a plane,' I say, as she has always said that nothing would get her 'up in one of those things.' Yet, Hayley and I still talk of trying to do something and we know boats would mean too many steps. 'You wouldn't go on a plane, would you?' I repeat.

'I would now.'

Amazement! This is a move forward, which is a miracle.

But my poor old thing, I think, it is probably too late now.
Her legs are bandaged, because of the cellulites, and I kneel at her feet stroking her legs.

'Don't' she snaps, 'people are looking.'

I drive away again, thinking of how she wanted me to stop smoking in that restaurant because I was upsetting strangers.

It is always me last. It is always my feelings, my offerings, that are rubbished, brushed aside. Lack of communication; that is one of my mother's problems I think as I arrive at my 'Sleeping Beauty' home, with the bushes nearly hiding the windows.

Somehow what is said to her always gets distorted. She certainly does not seem to hear the good, and what she wants to say gets muddled up even before it comes out of her mouth, probably even before it gets out of her brain.
Somehow she cannot get her messages out, or she is in the wrong place at the wrong time. Perhaps it is some genetic, some inherited thing, which ails her. In her veins maybe flow the memory cells of a noble woman who was never allowed to express an opinion, who never needed to think for herself, and so has never had the opportunity to gain real communication skills.

Whenever she went to visit a doctor, particularly when we were children, she was rarely clear about describing symptoms, never listened to his advice. Somehow I picked up from her ramblings that what she told the doctor was that her children never went to any parties and never got any parcels. I experienced this first hand when I went with her to some office to do with her council rent.

She had a query over the payments, and it took me a long time to get to the bottom of the problem. Mother kept on to the man about having no holidays! She was not telling the right people about her children's deprivations, and even if she did there would be no state department that was going to give her the money for parties and parcels or holidays.

If other mothers had invited us to their children's parties, could Mother have got us tidied up for them, and would she have bought and wrapped a present ? She certainly would not have held parties for us in return. We had no relatives who were likely to send us parcels. We sent none ourselves, so why would we expect any? Again I suppose what I was seeing was the ghosts of all the ladies who would have been used to wealthy uncles and godparents – would have servants to arrange parties and would expect to be invited everywhere.

If only she had had one good friend, just one who might have encouraged her to hold parties, perhaps run joint ones with her, and then the invitations would have come flooding in. The two could have scheduled to send each other's children inexpensive presents in the post. Maybe that would have been all she would have needed, a friendly ear to listen, someone to whom she could explain about the parties, the parcels and the holidays, instead of blurting it all out to a doctor and a rent officer, who could not be expected to provide such things.

I did arrange one holiday for her in recent years, through Social Services, but she didn't enjoy it much. It was the best on offer, and if I had said she needed to do it herself, she would have claimed not to know how to go about it. The comfort and attempt at helping that she received from me, was so often rejected. When I asked her what was wrong, or stroked her legs, I was spurned, and I think now I know why.

She could never let it be seen that she was accepting help, accepting kindness, for then I might think that she was all right. I might think I had no need to do anything for her anymore. Worse, I might leave her, might be free to be me, to pursue my own life, be freed from my victim role. For whatever happens, I have to stay in my role as it is the only way she can forget that it is she who is the greater victim, or forget her own abuse, or forget whatever other horror.

My telephone is ringing. It is Hilary, my clothes and jewellery lady, and she sounds distraught. 'I have told you about Agnes, haven't I?' She blurts out in a rush.

'Wasn't that your baby sitter, when your children were small?' Yes, I remember her, and I know Hilary still sees her. I was at Hilary's house once and she was giving the older lady some of her unsold clothes.

'Didn't you say that she was ill?' I ask.

'Yes she is in hospital now; I have been to visit her, bringing her washing home, taking in things she wants. You know...'

'So what is the matter?' Hilary sounds so upset.

'She was hurling sexual obscenities at me.'

'Sexual words? Sexual abuse?' I say in shock.

'Everything. Don't you see? All those years I left her in charge of my children.... I trusted her.' I try to calm my friend, my mind racing. She is confirming what I have been telling everyone all the time, ever since I began examining my mother, that illness strips away the pretences.

Hilary's baby sitter is an unmarried woman of great age, almost certainly a virgin. So what would eighty years of longing be like if it took that long to come out? Hilary is not to be comforted. She feels guilty about leaving her children with a woman she thought was respectable and is now acting as though depraved.

I do my best to reassure her and put the telephone down, wondering why Hilary should feel guilty. How was she expected to know? I wish women were not burdened with so much guilt.

*

I feel the guilt now, fear and guilt, and certainty self-doubt. I have been getting regular telephone calls from the Home over the last week as Mother's physical state begins to cause more alarm. The months have gone by and I am increasingly exhausted with hopeless hope about my Mother's life, and about my own. Imogen's first baby has been born and I have only seen her twice. I have not bothered to tell Mother and I feel I have always given her too much of my time to her, at the expense of my children.

I booked a Tupperware party six weeks ago, and it is today. Mother is now totally immobile, and is refusing to eat. But I did not panic or consider cancelling the party until last night, when I got news of yet another fall, this time out of bed. They are putting cot sides up, but will her body survive yet another bashing?

Only yesterday afternoon I was there trying to get her to eat her dinner, with no success. No to the cassette tape, no to the video, no to the dinner. I notice she is wearing a jacket like Anna's, like the one she envied on my daughter's last visit. I learn that Hayley managed to find one for her somewhere.

We sit in her bedroom as she does not want to get out of bed, but she had insisted on being dressed for me. As I look at the jacket and Rafe's gift of the tiny radio lying on her pillow, I think of my children being without a grandmother of the real kind. Should I tell her Imogen has a little girl?

Maybe a 'real grandmother' is the stuff of story books, but the gap between Mother's receiving and expectations, and her giving, is exceptionally wide.

Certainly there is a gap between my compassion for her and hers for me. For seeing the jacket, remembering Anna wearing it, brought back my eldest daughter's wedding. I was in the middle of my degree at the time, and in a relationship which, among other things, could be termed exhausting. The wedding reception ended late afternoon and Mother began whingeing that she could not go home yet, she would feel 'left high and dry,' so could she come back with me?

Gordon spoke to her, asking her if she had no empathy. I told him that he knew she hadn't, and I let her stay. It was not as though she wanted us, or company, because she took herself off to the end of my garden, enjoying the late afternoon sun and leafing through a magazine, looking smug, while I lay on the sofa exhausted, unable to move.

Would she give up a party for me, I think, as I get the room ready. Valerie told me recently that she had stood in the pouring rain that week, waiting for a bus to take her to see Mother in the Home, and saying silently in her head, 'you would not do this for me.'

I clear spaces on the top of the bureau and on my piano, and clear the table itself. As many flat areas as possible are needed to lay out the Tupperware goods. The first time I did this, the girl demonstrator expressed pleasure and almost surprise, especially when she saw that I actually had a table.
'Doesn't everyone?' I asked, surprised.

'No. The best one girl could do was an ironing board. People eat in front of the telly now, on coffee tables and trays.' I move the chairs from near the table and set them around the walls. I'm expecting quite a crowd, but I should not be having a party. Last night I telephoned the Home and asked them if I should cancel my party, I also called all my friends and Tessa the demonstrator. Would they rather not come? I might be called away, could they manage on their own if anything happened?

Churchfield House stressed that I must carry on with my life. My friends said not to worry as they would manage everything, and lock up for me, if I had to go. I am getting out the coffee cups when I hear the first knock on the door. Tessa is a young girl and very jolly and I know we will enjoy her chatter as she shows us how the Tupperware seals work, and all the newest lines.

Later, as with the jewellery, everyone has made their purchases and we are putting out the quiches and salads for the bring-and-share lunch. Apart from the venue, and organising the event, I provide only the basics like coffee and bread. These days are heaven for me since I get to keep all the leftovers.

'Is there any news on your agency lark? Sylvia asks.

'Nobody wants to meet me,' I joke. But really, no-one yet has interested me.

'Aren't you being a bit fussy? Linda suggests. 'We've have had this new woman join my water aerobics class. She is in her fifties, late fifties actually, and she answers advertisements from newspapers, Goes out with a different man every week.'

'Every week?' We all ask.

'Goes out? What – has sex?'

'Too right! Then, after a week she gets fed up with him, and calls the next one on the list.'

'I think she's lying,' I say

'Why do you say that?'

'Because I don't believe that so many men would be interested in a woman of that age. Most of them want a woman of thirty or even less, whatever their own age. You should see what I have been sent, all older than me, some seventy.'

'Well, maybe her men are seventy.'

'Would they all be up to it?'

'No of course not, I think she is lying to save her face.
Nobody likes to think they don't have a chance anymore.' try to explain that pride comes into it, something to do with having a sexual image I suppose. Nobody surely likes people knowing that they are starving. I hate it, but I cannot lie.

It would be great to parade myself as having a secret lover, or two, I could hold my head up and know that in the world's eye at least I was a desirable woman. I think a lot of women do just that, but I can't, and acting the lie would not change my burning frustration. I think of Bernard who admits to feeling lost and alone, whilst the old ladies pretend that they are in their busy pasts. I can't live a lie. Anyone at all close to me knows that I am without, and that I do mind.

'But why don't you go out with any man? Anyone from the list sent? They can't all be that unacceptable? If you are as desperate as you say you are.'

'Because I have to fancy them that is why. It simply would not work for me... What I dream of is a younger man.'

'So you want to be seen with a toy boy?

No, I am not interested in how I am seen. It's what I am doing that matters to me. Not to 'be seen' going out with men when I'm not, or when it is not good. No, I want a younger man because woman last longer than men, and so does their sexuality.'

'I still think you want too much.'

'Okay, so I settle for the eighty year-old who pops off in two years, or else the sixty year old who can't do it,' I laugh. 'Or do I go for the forty year-old?'

'And you still think that sex is the bottom of your mother's misery? No sex? When she was married and had four children?'

'What kind of activity does it take to make a child?'

Yes, I think, having had a poor sex life could well be the root of a lot of old age dementia. I tell them how it is recognised now that Alzheimer's is not always that. It can't be proved until after death, but what was thought to be the disease is now believed more often to be depression.

'...and what is depression? Sylvia asks, 'but plain old fashioned unhappiness.'

'And what causes that in old-age?' I question.

'Fear of death, I would say,' replies Tessa.

'Not being able to get out and about, do things anymore.'

'Not being useful.'

'Yes, okay, all of those, but you know, decades ago, I got a kind of intuition. After observing people I decided that when people are horrible it must be because they are miserable, and what they are often miserable about is likely to do with sex, or rather the lack of it. It is supposed to be the greatest pleasure available to man after all, and if you've never had it good – well, when you get old...'

'Why do you assume they've missed out?'

'Because a lot of us do, let's face it, be honest about it. How much real education do we get about sex to make it really good, to make it satisfying? Never mind bring the ecstasy claimed for it? Men I've been with have never wanted to be told what I want.'

`Yes on my wedding night,` one new guest speaks for the first time, ` it felt like my husband was on page one of the manual. Then page two. Then that was as far as he got.'

'You've just reminded me,' says Naomi. 'When you said about the men who might not be able to do it. I had a man once, for a very short time. It was ages ago, and he could only have been a bit over forty, and he couldn't do it at all. The first two times we tried,' she laughed, 'the only two times. He used to come and stay with me when I was on my own with the children. I had a spare bedroom in those days. Next time he came, I put him in there, but he didn't like it.'

'Why did you have him there at all if it was never any good? Why get as far as having him stay at all?'

'Because he was on business trips, that's how it all started. I was a useful stop off.... He was married too. But you see I couldn't take the disappointment. I could not take the being in bed and being all ready and perhaps the evening beginning.... Well and then... No it was better to be without than to have that.'

On my own, clearing up afterwards, planning to check out with the Home and then do some writing, I think so that is it. Women are dubbed not interested, frigid even, but really it is that their partner is impotent or cannot satisfy them. They give up on it, call it `that nasty business,' but then caress their own bodies and speak of something to remember. The bitterness of disappointment, could that be what sours, even drives one to madness?

Chapter 33

'You must ring Uncle Ernest,' Mother's voice sounded urgent and frightened. 'You ought to ring Uncle Ernest,' said Mother on the eve of my second marriage, ten years ago. had barely known the man five months and I was about to marry him in a month's time. 'You need someone to talk to, before you do this.'

Yes, I did indeed need a senior member of the family, an elder statesman as it were – if I had one. Ernest was Mother's oldest brother, and therefore the oldest on that side of the family, and since my father had no older relatives, and he himself was long dead, then I guess Uncle Ernest should have been the one I went to for fatherly support and advice.

But he never was a figure in my life. I hardly ever saw him. I knew his wife, Millie, better and her children, Elaine and the two boys, but we had gone forty years with little contact, until that time I saw Elaine and one of her brothers at Mother's hospital bedside.

Maybe Ernest was at work on the few occasions Mother took us to see Auntie Millie for we did not visit very often. If relatives lived far away many families hardly saw each other, for poor families could not afford train tickets. The only thing I remember about Uncle Ernest is him calling me 'Fat Pat.'

Why was my mother sounding so disturbed about my imminent marriage? I took no notice. She had never shown any concern for me. I did not value her opinion or judgement, either, so... why take any notice?

In fact I already had doubts about the man, but I wanted a relationship, and believed it would all be right once we were married.

I remembered now the first time Mother met him. We took her out on her Sunday treat together, took her for a pub meal, and she sat opposite him dropping food out of her mouth. Was she trying to scare him off? To me it seemed she was saying to him, you won't want to have a mucky old woman like me in your life. Just as she knew how to get through to doctors and social welfare departments in her frenzied telephoning and hospital days, she cleverly knew what to do. For that man was Mister Up-Market, Mr Fuddy Duddy, into appearances, and had no compassion for the old or afflicted.

But what she did not know was that he would have put up with anything at that moment before we were safely married and his money linked with mine in a joint owned house. The messy old woman in front of him in that pub could be ignored for the moment because of what he thought he was going to get out of me. She could always be dumped afterwards, neglected, abandoned, put into Residential Care before she needed it.

Great shame that I do not have a mother I trusted, for I would then have been warned off and spared eighteen months of abuse, followed by two years of an abusively run legal case. I never thought she had my interests at heart, and so took no heed. I thought that she simply did not want to share my attentions with him. For how many times had I gone to her and the cock had crowed? When I told her about my father in my bed, she simply snapped. 'Well, that's it. I'm leaving him now,' shaking her head from side to side and touching her hair as she always did.

'Did you know Dad has been married before?' that was what she said next. It was only how the news affected her, and just what kind of person he was, nothing about me. End of subject. Then I got mixed up with a boy when I was still at school and had an abortion. That was not legal at the time, but my doctor gave me pills because he knew of my home and family circumstances. I did not tell Mother until I was in my forties, and all she said then was that she thought school had told me all about that sort of thing.

Later, when I was going through yet another time of relationship break-up and depression, I sat with her in my house, over coffee, and told her about my life. About how all the put-downs had led to a low esteem, which just brought about more abuse. The next day she telephoned me.

'You know all you were saying to me yesterday? Were you trying to ask me for some money?'

I knew then that she had not heard what I was saying at all, not understood. I should have known, for once when she did read more, I passed on to her a book I had just finished. knew that she liked the author and that type of story, but I was nervous because the mother and daughter relationship in it was painful, and not unlike ours. I tentatively asked her how she was enjoying the story and in various ways tried to bring up the relationship problems, but in the end she just said, 'Is there something that worries you about this book?'

Perhaps I should have answered, but the very fact that she asked that and did not seem at all disturbed herself, told me that she was not picking up what the book was about. Or what could possibly be wrong with her for me.

But what role model did she have of family help? What extended family support did any of us have? My mother undoubtedly would have been affected by this lack. We only have to think of her first pregnancy and her years of child rearing with little money and a husband who was made to work long hours for years, 'living in' all week in my grandmother's paper shop..

For me there was more than a lack, there was a decided neglect. There was a positive aim to bring her down.
According to her relatives, she was 'put down' by her brothers from an early age. Then there was the harrying of my father to work in the shop for my grandmother, when he really wanted to do something else, so putting my mother into the very life she had wanted so desperately to escape . Add to that the keeping of my father at the shop night and day for the working week until Victor was eleven and Gordon one, leaving a woman to cope alone with children in a post war London.

I can't help believing that Uncle Albert, in particular, felt put out by having a working mother, who was also the dominant character in his household. For a man of this era, that might well have been unbearable. It almost certainly knocked his self-esteem. He stayed at home and worked in what was his mother's business for the rest of his life. So he took it all out on the only other female in the house.

Then I appeared, another girl who from an early age was clearly going to be another able woman. He could not bear it: killing Snow White then finding she had a sister – and so did what he could to flatten me. I remember him and his wife getting me on my own and haranguing me because my mother was 'lazy' and did not keep us children clean and tidy.

I remember, in my adult years, him ringing me from time and time with news of some death in the family, usually an old aunt I had never heard of. Using me, as my mother had no phone, but never asking how I was.

And if I had said I was having it hard with four children and little money he would have told me to get off my backside and go to work. For that is what he did say when I was studying to get into University and even with paper rounds, baby sitting and weekend jobs could still have done with help towards major clothes items like a winter coat or shoes.

When I passed the examination to go to Grammar School, I didn't get a bike as other children did, or even praise. I was a nuisance because I had to be bought expensive school uniform. My mother sold her ring, given by her Auntie Nellie and my father and Uncle Albert took me to buy what I needed.

'You'll have to work hard now,' Albert glowered at me. He was a man who was about work, about life having to be hard. Mother told me that if ever Dad complained about his long hours, Albert would insist that he had to 'work hard.' It was not as if by working harder Dad would earn any more money. To me, it felt as though he was saying that one had to work hard, not for betterment, but just to justify any kind of existence.

(Not him of course. He worked for profit and a far better life than my dad or any of us had.)

Maybe he was saying that to my dad because he had got Albert's sister pregnant, but I think it was more to do with guilt. Albert knew he had prevented my dad from getting a good job, just to ensure the misery of his sister, and he was making my father the scapegoat. When my mother was widowed at sixty, he told her to get a job, working in a factory, and when I challenged him on this, he told me that he thought she would enjoy it. I remember thinking that he didn't know his sister at all.

And he did scotch it all for me – the grammar school chance. He did it via my University grant. My friend, who was studying history and economic history, had already told me that my father was the lowest paid kind of worker in the land. So I expected to get a full grant, as she did with a builder for a father. But I found I was to get less than her.

There were all sorts of pressures on me as I got ready to go to University, and one was that I felt, as the lucky one of the family who had `got away`, I had to bring presents home every vacation. Money was worry enough but, finding the reduced grant I was to get, helped to finish me off. There were other reasons why I stayed at college for only a few days, but this was one of them

Why did I get a reduced grant, albeit having won an Open Exhibition? Because my father had to fill in on the forms that my mother received a wage. She did not, but Albert claimed, on his Income Tax forms, that he paid his sister a considerable amount of money each week to sort the greetings cards in his shop!

I wonder what would have happened if I had written to him and asked for that so called wage to be given to me for use at University? But I would never have done that, was not so programmed to look after my interests, and would have been stopped from doing it by my father, just as he stopped me signing the Petition to save Ruth Ellis from hanging.

When Albert died he left a little money to my mother and to both my brothers, but nothing to my sister or me. He even left nothing to Elaine, his niece, who lived near him and had looked after her father, Albert's brother, and then Albert himself.

I believe that he did not like woman and set my mother on her downward slope towards a very poor self-image, which then destroyed her life and, through her, mine too. At the time of Ernest's death, Gordon took me and my mother to the funeral, which began at Albert's house.

'What're you like at making coffee?' He asked as soon as we arrived from a long journey. As I thought that he must have things to do for the funeral, or perhaps had a bad leg, I made the coffee. However I soon discovered that there was nothing the matter with him, and he had nothing to do. It was his way of making his statement: that women are lesser and are the rightful servants.

During the day of the funeral, I overheard him telling someone that my mother was always saying, 'Poor Pat,' and that he wondered why she said that. If he wondered, then why did he not ever ask her about me? If he had known would he have helped me, with money, with an honest solicitor, with a boost to my self-esteem? Or would he have said that I should get off my backside and go out to work?

Why did Mother want me to go to her family for support when she had never received any from them herself? As the years go by I think of the wider family, I think of Mother's life.

*

Christmas passes, and since Imogen's baby, Lizzie has arrived I have been to see them in Wiltshire twice. My article 'Married, Dead or Deviant' has come back from two newspapers.

Mother swings from accepting her mother is dead, to believing that she is still in the old shop and she should go home to her. When she is acknowledging her mum is dead she says that my brother Gordon is working in the shop. Not only has he been 'a brick' and made all the arrangements, but he now runs the shop.

I ask her what about his teaching and she just snaps that he can do both jobs. Sometimes when she accepts the death she also accepts that the shop has gone. Then she says, 'Mum always said she would leave the shop to me.'

'I understand Mum now,' she says to me, something new. 'I understand Mum going in the shop all the time. She had to. It was her only social life. She could not get out much. She had broken her arm, you see.'

'I thought it was because she was fat,' I say. I can remember my grandmother on crutches, but the only cause I know was that she was enormous, and that was partly due to water retention. I still drink my two pints of water a day. The subject of her mother's inability to walk without crutches, which kept her housebound, is dismissed. Mother stays with the fantasy of the broken arm which was never properly healed, and that it was all her fault because her mother slipped and broke her arm running back to baby Nellie left alone in a bath.

Now I am getting more urgent telephone calls from the Home. Mother is now totally immobile and not eating. She may have to be moved to a Nursing Home.

So today I am at the meeting with all the usual officials, but no other family members. Mother needs nursing care and they do not have the nurses here. She is now completely and doubly incontinent. 'Is she likely to die soon?' I ask.

'Your mother is very tough,' they say. But she is refusing to eat, and they are finding it almost impossible to get her to take her medication. 'She hits the Carers,' I am being told.

I sit with her a while after the meeting. I am here later in the day than usual, because a late afternoon appointment was the best they could arrange at short notice, getting all the officials here.

'At least the evenings are light,' I say.

'It won't be long now, before they start drawing in,' says Mother. I remember this conversation I have had with her all my life. How she hates it when the evenings 'draw in,' how she hates the dark nights. We are already into June, it won't be long now.

'Why?' I have asked year after year. 'Why do you say that? What do you mean?'

'I don't know. When I was a child I hated it. It makes me depressed.' I try again to get her to say more, but all she ever says is that a dark sky and particularly the darkening sky of evening, has always given her a horrible feeling.

The sky is quite dark now, a storm has been forecast, and the Carers switch on the lights, and I remember how, when I lived at home, Mother always stood out against turning on the lights for as long as possible, so we sat in near darkness half the evening. She would not close the curtains either, not until very late. She said she did not like the lights turned on or the curtains drawn, because that meant the day had ended and was over.

'Oh don't turn on the lights yet. Don't shut the curtains. Don't shut out the day,' her sad, sad cry.

This is one of those where she believes Mum is still in the shop, and her request to me today is that I get her a spiritual healer. She wonders if one of the healers from her old church could help her to get home.

'Were you happy at home? I ask. 'Did your mother love you?'

'Of course she did. She spent a lot of money on me.'

'Tell me about the spiteful nuns.' I change the subject. I know that time is running out and I don't have all I need to know, to understand my mother.

'They are crafty, she tells me. 'They used to creep about. They had nice smiley faces. But then they would make you work hard.' I have never been able to get her to say more about the nuns. The meeting and the talk with Mother has taken up a lot of my time. I tell her I have to go, and stand up quickly, hoping that it is clear I will accept no delaying tactics.

'You ought to grow your hair,' she calls out as I walk away.
'You ought to grow your hair and have a perm. Then you might get a nice man.'

As I drive away, I am tense with so much to do running round in my head. I have been given the names and numbers of various Nursing Homes to ring. They want Mother moved as soon as possible and they also advised me that I should view all the possibilities first. I am working on a novel, and I could do with giving the house and garden more attention. There is a man, whose details have come from the agency, and I would like to make contact.

The pressure mounts as I turn the car into my drive, and as I go indoors I find that the telephone is ringing. Mary from the church, she of Greek book reading fame, is calling to say she has a tape for me. She had a slight heart scare recently, and the hospital gave her a tape, designed by the medical world, to relax heart patients. She has told me about it before, and now says she has made a copy of it for me. I tell her I would love to have it.

For so long I have wanted to make everything all right for my mother. I worked hard at school so that one day I could take her round the world, and I have conducted more and more of her business as she has grown older, accompanied her to look at flats, to see officials, see doctors. Even when she went into a Residential Home, I did not give up hope of finally bringing her some happiness. I asked both her Homes if she could go on holiday and was told that it would be too disturbing for her. Hayley and I have racked our brains to think of ways of getting her abroad.

Gordon and I did take her out of the Home, to the seaside, a couple of times. I recall now how scared we were the last time because she looked as though she were about to breathe her last, so we took her back early. As I left her that day, she looked into my face and said, 'I put you down as a cruel person,' because I had shortened her outing.

I have hoped that an old man would come into the Home and be her lover. Mother has had no fulfilment in any way, and right up until now I have hoped to somehow bring her to joy.

For some time now I have wanted, but not had the energy, to arrange, that an Aromatherapy Masseur go regularly to Churchfield House to give my mother massage treatment. I had hoped that being touched and rubbed with oils, might produce some effect of sexual sublimation, and I wanted that massage to be accompanied by soothing music. Now all I can hope for her is that she reaches some kind of serenity, some kind of inner peace, and perhaps Mary's tape will have that effect.

The next day the tape arrives and I take it to the Home. I have to go again so soon, because they told me when I was there yesterday that Mother is nearly out of cash. There is nothing left in the funds they keep for her to pay for her Daily Mirror and hairdresser, should she still want those things. I do not have the time to go to her bank, and I can only take what little cash I have in my house. As always, when I get these urgent requests, they are often quite sudden. What little money I have will have to do until I next go to Kingston.

After an extensive search in the Home, none of us can find the cassette machine, which one of the Carers got for me and that Mother has never used. I go into the office and take in the cash. I shall need to get more money, but when will I ever get to the bank in the next few days?

Driving home, I think of the difference between me and Mother in our handling of money. I run my car by cutting open toothpaste tubes, using old envelopes, which I stick with sellotape, and by washing out sauce and jam jars to flavour soya stews.

Once, on one of the Sunday outings, I paid for lunch and everything. It was Mother's Day and that was my gift to my mother. The next week I asked her what she had done with the money saved, the money she would normally have spent on the day. She did not know. Well, she was always accused of being a fritterer. That gift had made no difference to her, but it would have made a huge difference to me. Oh, how I would have made that ten pounds work for me!

Back home, I call one Nursing Home after another, only to be told they have no vacancies. I call another, and they too have no spare bed either, but would I like to come and view, in case a place becomes available. I will be bringing Molly home from school for the rest of the week, so it is impossible.
I call another Home and they have a vacancy, but the only time I can visit to view is tomorrow at three, Molly's time. accept the place anyway.

Later Imogen telephones me, the new baby Lizzie, is fine. We chat for a while. She is back in her teaching post, but will break up a week before her husband does. He is a Maths teacher in a different school. Can she come to stay for those few days with the baby? I am delighted. She is the only one of my children who does not live near me.

After the meditation, instead of my book, I read again the few sentences describing the man from the agency. He sounds exactly what I have been looking for. It will soon be sleep time, but I have to leave my nightly read, because of doubts about my hasty decision in accepting the Nursing Home. I have never seen it. I ring my youngest brother, my sister and one of my daughters, and ask if they could manage to get away at three tomorrow to view the Home? No. Churchfield House won't keep Mother much longer, so she will have to go to the only place which has a definite vacancy, which I have no time to view. Anyway, it is the only one in a road which I know how to get to. Although in Ewell, it is on a familiar route.

Today I go to Churchfield House and inform them of my decision. They tell me that I will have to pack up her things. The last Home did this for me, when she moved. They have found the tape machine, but it is not working. I go home to write, call friends, and do some exercises until it is time to collect Molly. Tomorrow I must fit in a swim.

The next day when I call the Home they have fixed the machine, but when I ask whether they have played the meditation tape to her, they do not know what I am talking about. I spend the morning writing, but instead of swimming I rush to the Home before it is time to collect Molly. We all search for the tape. Mother is in bed. She is looking very frail, and asking to go home.

After Molly and my soya meal, I sit quietly listening to Mozart's Requiem before beginning my meditation routine. Tomorrow I have to pack all Mother's belongings and clothes, before going for Molly again. Maybe there will be time somewhere in the day for a swim. Then there is writing and the weekly vacuuming. I want to go to the library and check the answers to a crossword I pinched from Bernard. I need to make a birthday card.

I did so want a full life for my mother. I wanted her to travel and to love me. I would have loved her to be sufficiently at peace to want more: to want to read, to draw, to add to her small knowledge of history and music. My mother was a woman sexually abused as a child, put down by family, caught up in a wrong marriage. A woman who had children she did not want and could not care for, because she had never been cared for herself and had no role model.

I suddenly recall how, when I was a young mother, Mother referred to her maternal days and told me that she had seen a programme on television where it was claimed that some animals reject their children. She said this with almost a glee, with something of a lip-licking smugness. Oh that's all right then, Mother, I thought, if some animals reject their young you are let off the hook.

So now there is little hope left of earthly happiness, but perhaps some of eternal, restful peace.

The only way Mother could cope with her own life being destroyed was to destroy me, and I read in my spiritual books that cruelty is inflicted because someone who suffers a great deal can feel better if they can watch someone else being tortured. Or did the books say that it helps them forget their own pain? Whatever the reason, there is hope for me still, and I must cling on to that. But as I study again the profile of the agency man, I think, do I really want to bother again? To make that effort, raise those hopes? Only to be disappointed, or worse, and end up like the last time.

Beautiful Dreamer

*

'What are you messing about at now?' Mother asks. 'They tell me I can go home any time I like.' It has taken me two hours to pack her clothes, shoes, photographs, radios, ornaments, bits of furniture, cosmetics and toiletries. I have to hunt for the footstool, which had found its way into the lounge.

There are postcards from various family members on holiday, and notelets from my friends wishing her well, some old Mother's Day cards and Easter ones. There is a new card from Hayley, saying that she is about to go away and hopes that Nanny will take care of herself, and be well in her absence. I cannot stay and listen to my mother's complaints any longer. I thought the packing would take half an hour, and I have missed my swim. But I did manage to call Mary last night and ask for a new copy of the meditation tape which I so wanted to play to Mother.

Mother is to be moved later on today. Thank goodness the Home is responsible for transferring all the medication. They did say that family is responsible for taking the client and her belongings, but since the only family that is likely to do it is me, I have told them that I am too busy. I say goodbye to the Carers, realising that this is the last time I will come to Churchfield House.

They will miss her, they say to me. I pop to the toilet near the entrance, and then say goodbye to the woman in reception. She will miss my mother too.

'But she is so difficult,' I say.

'Ah, but she has such a beautiful smile,' she tells me.

And, oh, what potential for happiness and love – and laughter – lies in that smile?

I grieve.

Chapter 34

It is my first visit to the Henley Nursing Home, and as I pull into the drive I see it is a large old house. The two previous Residential Homes were purpose built, bright and modern, and they were financed by local councils, but Nursing Homes are nearly always privately owned.

The day Mother arrived I had a telephone call from this new place explaining that the previous one had not sent all the medication. I would have to go there, collect it and take it to them. I said no, so I do not know what they did. It is interesting that I do and do and do, and then suddenly draw in my horns. It must be a syndrome similar to that seen in my mother, of opposite behaviours, see-sawing.

I am met at the door by the Manager, who leads me into what seems to be, from the size of the building, the only living room. The residents sit round in a large circle, their chairs touching, and a television set as their only focus. They do not look at it, but loll and dribble and shout.

Then I see my mother. She is on a hoist. I assume they are moving her from her chair to a wheelchair. But no, she is being wheeled out of the room on the hoist. This can't be right. I follow the nurses attending her and find them going into what must be her bedroom. It is small and I can see there will not be enough room for all her things. There is one small cupboard and a large window ledge, and that is all the space for things, not enough for all the photographs, cards and ornaments, or any flowers she might receive.

'Why are you moving her like this? I ask. 'Why do you not take her in a wheelchair? They are taking her off the hoist, and easing her into the only chair, and explain that it is safer this way. There are fewer moves at which she could be dropped if they do only chair to hoist to chair. Far more risky, they claim than the procedure I expected of chair to hoist, hoist to wheelchair, wheelchair to hoist, hoist to bedroom chair.

I start to stow her belongings as best I can. Maybe the rest I will have to take away. Another day I will go through everything with her, and see what she wants to keep most. As I work I remember another time of unpacking in a Residential Home. It was when Mother went to a local Home for a week's Respite Care, some years before she became a permanent resident. We were taken to her bedroom by a Carer who then instantly, without a word, opened up Mother's small hold-all and began putting things into cupboards and drawers.

'Do you have to do that? Mother asked. She did not sound very hopeful, sounded resigned as she so often did. And no doubt she felt exposed seeing her tatty old garments being pulled out and seen.

'It's just what we do, unpack for people coming in.'

'She would prefer to do it herself,' I said.

Where did that come from? I wonder. Why do I sometimes, so rarely, know exactly what to say? Like Mother who could be so timid when so often she is belligerent, I who also seem never to find my voice, occasionally find myself standing up to something.

Thinking of that now, how Mother did not want her unpacking done for, I am reminded of her asking for her clothes to be changed several times a day. Oh, what little control older or disabled people have over their lives. No wonder they insist on small victories.

Mother is now banging on the little table that has been placed across her chair, like a television meal table.

'You have made it worse,' she says to me, looking straight into my face.

Well, everything is always my fault, isn't it? My brother and I both took her home early from the sea. But it was I who got called cruel.

I carry on working. There is nowhere for me to sit anyway.

Her words have aroused all the old anger in me, but I am also filled with horror and pity, and even more anger at the sight which met me on my arrival, seeing my mother perched there on the hoist. She was being dragged along on the hoist, looking like a monkey on a stick, and the look on her face was the one that was really always there, even beneath the snarling anger and bitter attack. It is the same look I saw when she was having her back bashed by my father, the same look when I saw her face covered with blood after falling when running for a bus, that look of resignation.

Was it always there, behind the nasty looks, the look that said, `Oh, isn't it a shame? Can't you afford to have your hair done? Can't you manage to get a holiday? Isn't it terrible?`
For that was Mother all my adult life. Yet when I did have it good, the tune was changed. When I got a dish washer, she told me not to tell my sister, in case she would be jealous. If I were going on holiday, it was 'aren't you lucky? Then of course I would feel bad because I was going on holiday and she was not. There was no weeping with those that do weep, no rejoicing with those that do rejoice, with Mother.

When I was only twenty-three, had a two year-old child and was pregnant, my husband became very ill, and nearly died. They never found out what it was, but at first they thought it was rheumatic fever. When I telephone my mother, from a call-box, to tell her my husband had rheumatic fever, she said, 'well I have always told you your house was damp!' She rubbed in your misfortunes and spoilt small joys. Yet I still feel that the real her, the bottom line, was the resignation, and maybe the bad behaviour was the only buzz – fun perhaps – she could get out of life.

Yet here I am yet again, her champion, fighting her fights.

I am disgusted at the sight of her on that hoist. It cannot be right, cannot be necessary for 'safety' purposes. I saw none of this in the two previous places. What about the dignity of the clients?

I have thought about it for the last few days, have spoken to the Manager on the phone, and here I am, at the new Home again to see him. But first I must visit Mother. Once again my eyes are met by the clients sitting, chair touching chair in a circle, drooping, dribbling and shouting, – degraded souls. Mother is banging on the little tray fixed over her chair.
Is that the last resort of the desperate? Do they feel they have to bang and protest?

It brings back to me one of the times when the man from Kingston Carers came to see my mother with me when she was still in her flat. We discussed her life, her problems, and it was at this interview that I finally spelled it out to her that she was never going to come and live with me. When the man left, I went to leave and she banged on her living room floor with her walking stick. 'Stay! Don't go yet. You stay with me a little while more.' Although not getting her way completely – or perhaps to her just not yet – she was proving to herself that she could at least still flex her bullying muscles.

And, of course, I did stay. But first I went with the man to the door of the block of flats, to thank him for his visit. When I came back to Mother`s flat, the room smelled. She had passed wind and it was stinking. Fear I thought – don't people shit out of fear? A terrible fear that she was losing control of me. For a moment I contemplated something worse. Evil. Don't some associate the devil with a smell of faeces? Could it really be that my mother`s attitude to me was evil intent?

This time she bangs with a knife. It must be a meal time, and sure enough, meals are being dished out. In the front of my mother is placed a plate of baked beans, a frankfurter sausage and a slice of bread and butter. One of the nurses tells me that she is still refusing to eat, so I try to feed her, but she either turns her head away as I approach with a forkful, or if I get it into her mouth she pushes the food out with her tongue. After a while of trying, she looks at me and says, 'you eat it.'

I would not actually mind, Mother. Free food. Me, who has always been so hungry. In every way.

There is something in me that is always warmed by the gift of food, free food, but it is a disgusting meal. I do my best, tell her I will be seeing her in a few days, and go off to find the Manager's office. What he takes me to is no more than a cubby hole. It reminds me of the Caretaker's office when I was at school, no more than a base for someone whose job took him out and around and who had minimal paper work, no telephone calls, and certainly no visitors. There is only one hard backed chair and he has to go hunting for another one for me to sit on while we talk. I am reminded of the plush offices, the easy chairs aplenty, of the trays of cups and saucers and milk jugs and sugar bowls and biscuits, at meetings in the past two Homes. I ask for a cup of tea, and he goes himself to get it, coming back with two mugs in his hands. The telephone rings twice while I am with him and he speaks at length. Where are the secretaries, the Carer's free to make tea?

First, I hand him the meditation tape, saying that I will play it to Mother the next time I come, but could he get the staff to try it for her between times? He takes it from me and says he will put it somewhere safe, and will tell the nurses about it. At last I have got it together, after lost tapes and broken machines. I first got the tape two weeks ago, but still have not played it to Mother.

We begin with the hoist, and the Manager again insists that the way it is used in this Home is perfectly in order. He also tells me that he is only here three days a week; that he is a part time Manager, and he lives in the West Country. I ask about the food, about activities, about visits by doctors, and he reassures me on all these issues. 'Do you have any outings? I ask. 'Any entertainments for the residents?'

'Oh yes,' he informs me, 'every month.' I am not convinced.

'And when is the next one? I ask.

He turns the pages back and fore in his desk diary. Back and fore, flipping the pages but hardly looking at anything. Suddenly he stops and looks up. 'Next Wednesday,' he says. But he does not bother to tell me what the entertainment is, or at what time.

The way he turned the pages seemed as though he was just going through the motions, and just stopped at a random page. I felt he was making it up, and he does not ask me to make a note of it. He does not show me the entry. It reminds me of when I asked my mother how long she was married before she had my brother, and what she wore as a bride.

Pretend answers. Glib, is that the word for both instances of hasty response? Or lies?

As I leave I ask to use the toilet. There is not one for visitors. I would have to go upstairs and use the residents' ones.

Driving home, I know that soon I will have to go through my mother's belongings. Involve her in decisions. Take things to the

Charity shops. Perhaps hand photographs and things out to family. I have put up the last card she received, the one from Hayley.

Back home, I prepare for a healthy, but tasteless cheap evening meal. I could do with playing that relaxation tape myself. Maybe Mary will make me another copy. After my meal, it is oiling, yoga, bath and finally my meditation. But will I ever heal Mother? Is it too late?

*

The following morning with meditation done, then general exercises, I breakfast on oats, boiled in water only, then I am off to my writers' group once again in Sylvia's house. There will be a bring-and-share lunch: quiches, cold meats, salads, cheeses, French bread, cake and wine. I can hardly wait. As I run the group for nothing, I seldom make a contribution.

At the beginning of each meeting, I give notices, new homework titles and we set the next date and venue of the class. After that everyone, hopefully, has something new to read, and if there is little material because hardly anyone has done their homework, then I have a few exercises up my sleeve and other ideas to resort to, like topics for discussion. Talking and sharing ideas is one of the best aspects of my group. It is my favourite part of any group I attend, and even social ones. I am good at getting a discussion going and my children have learned it through me. At the writing class something usually comes up as a result of a story or article, but if not I read something, quote something, bring up an issue that is dear, or funny, to me – anything which will get people going, and preferably heatedly.

Today I bring up the subject of my mother not eating, and I get the usual response that this is the way old people have of telling you they want to die. I don't like that idea, don't believe it, and fill the group in on my thoughts regarding age and our misconceptions about it. I tell them that dementia, senility, Alzheimer's disease are, in my view, all useful terms to label old people as mad. For if they are mad, they are beyond us, and we do not have to do anything for them, and certainly not for their inner state. I remind them that it has been proven that Alzheimer's is rarely that. Experts now believe that the symptoms we see, and give the name to, are often caused by depression.

Depression we could perhaps help, but does anyone have the time or the inclination? How much tolerance do we have for that in someone whatever their age?

'Oh I think they have just had enough', says Sylvia.

'My mother has certainly not had enough, not of life. Not of its good things.'

'Had enough of the bad things then? Mike says, the only man in the group.

'And want to go when that is all they've had?' I ask. In recent years when I have felt suicidal, what has stopped me is anger that what I have had is all I am ever going to get.

'Don't want to go on into more old age and illness and feebleness,' says the oldest member of my class.

'Don't want to hold on to hope?' I ask, remembering Mother looking as though she were gasping to stay alive in the hope that one day she would have a life.

'Oh, come on, at eighty – what's your mother, ninety? They've had a good innings,' two speak at once.

'My mother has had no innings.' I say angrily for once.

I used to say that I did not want anyone ever saying of me that, that I had a good innings. When I came out of the last divorce I felt I had had no innings at all! It felt like my lawyers were working for the other side and, as I tried to fight all alone, people kept telling me to get on with my life and I replied that I did not have a life.

Of course it is better now. I have my children and my friends. My fifties in fact have been my best years: with classes and cinema and coffees out – and friends. But the phrase ` gets on with your life` is a stupid and unkind one to make to anyone in distress. There is more than one way of getting on with it, and if you are still alive you are doing that.

My life in those early days was to react to, and try to get justice for, that awful divorce.

I never got justice, but I have survived and, in recent years, have come to love my house. It could even be said I have achieved a reasonable innings. But not a sexual one.

Mother took herself out, so she did make a bit of a life. I am luckier in that my inclinations led me, not to lonely outings, but to people.

Bringing my head back to the class, I hear they have moved on to the subject of euthanasia I tell the class what I heard on the radio, a programme about that. A doctor who worked in a hospice said that, in his experience, the patients who came there wanted to live out their lives whatever it was, be it weeks or days.

'So why do you think that some old people spit out their food? Sylvia asks.

'I suppose most of us have always seen that as a statement of not wanting to be kept alive,' Mike answers.

'Yes,' Christine, a new member, remarks thoughtfully, 'but we do like to tidy things up don't we? Label things and people. Tidy the old way.'

'Call someone demented rather than look at what might be behind their behaviour? Say they want to die, when not eating is something else?' I throw out for consideration.

'I sometimes think we don't want to see the old, or the mad, because it reminds us of what we might become,' says Mike.

'Do we say that they want to die and encourage them to let go?' Christine says.

'You know,' Sylvia looks thoughtful. 'I thought when I was very young that the old became so unattractive, so wrinkled and sunken and hollowed eyed, so that we didn't mind them going. But a baby is so pretty, always, whatever it turns out to be later. There is something gorgeous about a baby, don't you think? Delectable even – think of what people say, ' oh I could eat him'. It is nature's way of making sure a baby is cared for and protected.'

'So what do you think this not eating is in your mother?' Several speak at once.

'I think it is one last claim – a common one – to have control over life. Someone washes them, changes their incontinence pads, chooses what they will wear, where they will sit, what time they will go to bed, and what they will eat. They have control over absolutely nothing.'

'Except not to eat? Not to swallow their pills?' Several speak at once.

'Even choosing to die?' I say.

'There you are then.' Sylvia says smugly.

'But it is not that they want to die. Don't you see? But if they know they are likely to die soon, then maybe the last little bit of power is to choose how and when. Maybe that is what motivates requests for euthanasia, just like someone's last act in their drama is written and staged by them. Not eating is saying look here, I am a person too. You do this and you do that for me, but you are not going to get away with thinking that I am one of those new dolls into which you can put some pretend food, so that you can change my pretend nappy.'

It is time to get on with the reading out of class members' own work. Then we eat and at the end of the meal there is some left over quiche which I am given to take home.

I can see my mother now, only in her seventies, opening her mouth like a baby bird as I fed her medicine with a spoon. There was something about the way her mouth opened, shaped itself, and the way her mouth and tongue closed around the spoon which I found unpleasant, almost obscene. It was as though she was feeding from my breast.

My sister always reminds me how, in very early days of Mother's widowhood, if she sat next to me on a sofa at a family party, she would put her head on my shoulder. It was as if she was saying, look at me with my mummy. I remember with equal pain how she snuggled into a coat I once held out for her. My lady's maid is dressing me. Or my mummy is dressing me. How often has she said lately that the last thing she remembers before coming into the Home was her mother putting on her coat? People talk to me of role reversal in old age, but Mother has never been a mother to me. Now I am supposed to mother her, my children, and my grandchildren, when I have no role model of mothering – or of being mothered – to follow.

I am going to have to fight concerning this business of the hoist, although no mother or mother figure fought for me when I went through my seemingly illegal divorce. No Affidavits. No Disclosure of Means.

So today is church. Mother has been in the Nursing Home for just over a week, and I will visit her as soon as I get home from Richmond. I have done my meditation early and even managed some writing. Sometimes I wake early and find it painful to lie in late, aching not to be in bed on my own. I leave on the bus with my bottle of water and book. I have my free bus pass now, so can go to church more often. Mother got hers soon after she was widowed, and I could feel her sense of lightness, her sense of being able to fly, anywhere. I was looking after her when she was that age, the age I am now.

I smile as I stand at the bus stop. There is a small local supermarket at the end of my road and it opens at ten on a Sunday. At five to ten, as I wait for my bus, already there is a queue for the shop. How could anyone want something that much, to come out too early and have to wait? It is not exactly Harrods' Sale, is it? Perhaps all these people do not like being alone in their beds too.

I read on the bus, a murder mystery, which I allow myself more of, in the break between literature class terms. After the service I am given a large bunch of flowers. Sunday's flowers are usually given to someone in need, and these are for my mother. I generally put off going home by going to a Burger King with Mary. It is the only place for a cheap snack since most of the places in Richmond do nothing other than large dinners. Mary has a burger with a cup of coffee, whilst I have only a small portion of chips. I will drink water on the way home, and have a cigarette when I get there, before I set off to see Mother with the flowers.

Chapter 35

I know. I really know it. As soon as I see Mother today, deep down I know she is dying. They explain that they have been trying to get in touch with me, and I find her in bed looking hollow and grey, but I am told the doctor is coming to see her.

She is groaning. She wants to go home. She does not care about the flowers I have brought from the church. I sit for a while and check the cassette player is working but the tape is lost again. The Manager is not in today, and the nurse does not know where he has put it.

I go with Esme, the senior nurse, and she hunts through some lockers. We hunt through my mother's things and Mother watches us. I stay the time I have allocated for this visit, then go home to write.

The guilt has mounted while I have been writing, and when I was washing out a jam jar to go in my soya curry. I call Imogen at six, as I always do on a Sunday, and we talk as we always do while we both cook. We plan what we will do when she comes to stay in a week's time. At seven I call the Home. The doctor has been and Mother has a respiratory infection. She has taken her medicine and is a lot better. 'She asked to go to the toilet,' Esme says, 'so I told her I would take her if she took her medicine. You have to use a bit of bribery.'

I have seen Carers ignore, or be snappy about, requests to go to the toilet. I don't blame them, they are all over worked, and I know how it was for me with a toddler wanting the potty when I was breast feeding a new baby. But what must it be like for the old person to be refused, and be forced to sit there and fill an incontinence pad? Bribery? We bribe with sweets and money and promises of love and affection, but that to be taken to the toilet should come down to being a treat!

'Will you move her back into the living room?' I ask, thinking of her alone in her tiny room, her lonely bed.

'Not until tomorrow.' Mother is a lot better. I put the telephone down at seven twenty. I spend some ten minutes turning off my computer and clearing up my study, then some minutes doing exercises.

Then I get a sudden urge to have something else to eat. I am in the kitchen putting butter and marmite on some toast, when the telephone rings.

'Is that Patricia?'

'Yes.' I can hear it is Esme.

'Brace yourself, Patricia. Your mother passed away ten minutes ago.' It is ten to eight now, so it must have happened at twenty to eight.

She went before the dark settled. It is summer. She went before that time when you draw the curtains and shut out the day. Before the coming of the dark and frightening sky.

'What happened? You only just put the telephone down. You told me she was better.'

'I looked in on her. Soon after talking to you. She looked white. We got the oxygen mask, but she went very quickly.'

Esme says she will call Victor and ask him to tell Valerie. I tell her I will telephone Gordon. I call Anna first. She will tell my other children, and Gordon. I call Vanessa, my Minister. We had planned to meet in Kingston tomorrow anyway, just for a coffee and a chat before my swim. Now it will have to be business. I call the Home. 'What happens now? Do they organise everything?'

'No, you have to do it.'

'But tomorrow? It can wait until tomorrow?'

'No. We can't keep her here. You will have to arrange it tonight.' I look through the telephone directory, the Yellow Pages, but I cannot find the number of the place nearest to me. Maybe I can't see because my eyes are spinning. I call Christine, new to the writing group, but already a close friend of mine. She lives around the corner from the place. She has the number in her Church magazine, and says it if is not right she will walk up the road and look at the door. I call the number she has given me. It is a central number for all branches anyway, and I could have found it in the books. I call Mary who was with me for lunch. I call Mike from the group as he has an answering machine so I know I can get through, but he is in, and says he will tell the rest of the group.

Rafe calls and says he will pay for anything I need to get through the next few weeks, whether it is taking a taxi to go swimming, or some treat or easy to cook food, even some booze, and I must get it and charge it to him. He describes a breathing exercise to do which will calm me.

I call the Home. The undertakers have just been for Mother. I fall asleep.

Early the next morning I am already at my computer. I have had a call from the Funeral Directors, which was full of charm, condolences, and professionalism. Now the telephone rings again and this time it is the Coroner. Again the condolences and he explains what happens next. He needs fuller details than the ones he has been given, like Mother's second name, and place of birth. We even chat about our separate relationships with our mothers. I am warmed, but panic when he says that the death has to be registered because it has to be done in a place I do not know how to get to. She died in Ewell, and the place for registration is in Epsom, in a part I do not know.

I am just heaving my rucksack of swimming things onto my back when Anna and her husband arrive to see that I am all right, and to tell me that they have not managed to contact my youngest brother. He is not answering his mobile or land line telephone.

I arrive in Kingston by eleven and meet Vanessa. We have a coffee and talk about the funeral arrangements, then about life, people and psychology. 'I'd like to go and see my mother,' I say, 'but I am scared.' I tell her that I won't go unless I can get someone to go with me, Gordon perhaps, or maybe my friend who lives around the corner from the place will come with me.

'I'll go with you,' Vanessa offers. She has seen many dead bodies, as she was a nurse before she trained to be Minister.

When I get home, the Coroner calls to tell me that he is not happy with the cause of death. The doctor in attendance diagnosed respiratory infection, but he was a locum, and my mother had only been moved there a few days ago. She had not been seen by her regular doctor from where she had been treated for the last two years, days ago. The Coroner regrets that there will have to be a post mortem. I tell him I am pleased, that in spite of her age she still matters, and that she is getting attention, which was what she always wanted.

When I put down the telephone, I laugh to myself. Mother is in the central Funeral Home in Kingston, now she will go to Epsom Hospital, then back to Kingston. Later, she will be brought to my nearest funeral parlour, and from there will be driven to Kingston Crematorium. Gadding about to the last.

And now I am skipping my meditation as I have been invited out by my actress friend to a fringe theatre in London. I am gadding about too.

The next morning I get a call from Hayley. Anna had sent her sister a voice mail with the news to her in Florida. Telephone calls from friends and relations wanting information, offering sympathy and, in the middle of it all, I run out to my corner supermarket and buy some gin and tonic and some halva, as well as a tin of vegetable chilli, courtesy of Rafe. Then telephone calls, meditation and more telephone calls. Anna has, at last managed to get hold of Gordon, but I do not hear from him.

On Tuesday afternoon I am at the keyboard when I get a call from the Funeral Directors, they want to know when I am coming in to arrange the funeral. It has to be done by Thursday. Wednesday I have arranged to collect Mother's belongings from the Home, and I have to sort through it all. Thursday I have Molly, then to drive some of the things to a Charity shop. From there, I have to drive to Tessa to pick up some Tupperware goods she wants me to deliver, and Imogen has sent me a list of things she needs for her new baby when she comes to stay next week. I will have to do it now. They can see me in twenty minutes. No time to get somebody to come with me.

*

'Burial or cremation? The very sweet lady is asking.

'Cremation,' I say, my mother was claustrophobic, hated being indoors. Always said that she wanted that, would hate to be 'down there.'

Will I want to view my mother? Yes? Then they will need photographs of her so that they can make her look as she looked in life, hairstyle and everything. I choose the very best of the coffins recommended for cremation. Poor old girl, she had no better dress all her life.

('I never had a dress worth more than five dollars,' said the woman going to her own funeral.)

And what will she actually wear? Do I want to bring in some item of Mother's clothing? I think of the gravy stained dresses and say no. They tell me they can supply a lovely white dress with a frill around the neck. 'Ever so pretty,' says the lady, as if it is going to matter, as if Mother is going to notice or object, and I think of the brown velvet dress and brown velvet bow.

The visit has taken an hour and a half. Late home, I run round the other corner and buy myself fish and chips – yet more thanks to my son. I am going to Christine's this evening for our monthly coffee and catch up on news and social things, which perhaps I should not be doing, but it was booked last month and, besides she lives near the funeral place so I will be able to drop off the photographs of Mother looking her best.

Wednesday, I change Mother's bank account to my name only. I will pay her expenses out of the remaining funds. She went into Residential Care heavily in debt because of the regular and frequent taxis and countless phone calls, which she needed to support her life when in the flat. Her pension has been used to contribute to her care, but a little was allowed for pocket money, and that has accumulated, a lot unspent. Poor old girl never had a penny in her life, and now pays for her own funeral. I collect her belongings from the Home and the Manager is there this time. It is only a week since I met him. He says he is very sorry for what happened, and helps me out to the car with the black bags. He also hands me the meditation tape, which, too late, has now been found.

But he has lost Mother's corner unit, the one from the friend she did like

I have a telephone call from the Coroner. Mother did not have a chest infection after all, but died of bronchial pneumonia, and she is now gallivanting back to Kingston.

The cards have started to come and I am surprised how much difference they make. Hayley, from Florida, writes, `I like to think that Nan is with her mum now.`

I discuss with my sister on the telephone where to have the reception then book it, and arrange the food.

The funeral people have asked about music. I have always known what one of the pieces would be. I have known it since the nurse said what she did about my mother's figure, and it includes words which echo what I hope – `then will all clouds of sorrow depart.`

Three pieces of music are required. In a way I already half know what I would chose. The song I heard her singing in the war, in the days of the knife at my brother's throat, but the third? Well she loved the Beatles, but which one? I finally speak to Gordon and suggest Eleanor Rigby because Eleanor was my mother's name, but he thinks the words are inappropriate. He is dealing with the registration, and I am relieved.

Vanessa rings me to say she will ring my mother's other children for anything they might wish to include in the funeral service. Immediately I put down the telephone, Imogen calls about her proposed visit. She had planned to come for a few days next week, but that week will end with the funeral on Friday. She has an appointment in Wiltshire on Thursday and does not want to make the journey twice in such a short time. I can understand that she cannot come up to London twice and that I have to choose to have her with me for three days, or have her at her grandmother's funeral. I ask if I can think about it.

I visit Linda from the Literature class to try on her three black dresses and take two away with me. The weather looks as though the dresses will be too hot.

Sitting with Molly, waiting for Anna to come home from school, I write the eulogy. My handwriting is in danger of becoming like my mothers, and Imogen begs that I type my weekly letter to her. But it is strange that I can always write legibly when I have to, like when I sit an examination, and I do it now. Writing quickly, in the half hour that I have, with an A4 lined pad balanced on my knees, I write a legible eulogy of which I am proud of.

Some of my friends say they will come next Friday. Those who can't, I ask to send flowers. I ask everyone to send flowers, and I ask people to send individual sprays rather than one collective one. I want the poor old girl covered, massed, with flowers on the coffin, around it, and on the top of it. She had so little in life.

All my life, Mother said that she did not want flowers when she died, she would rather have a cup of tea in someone's house. Well, she did not get much of that. She was a loner, did not have a lot of friends, and would not have reciprocated with a cup of tea in her home because she did not want to tidy it up. She did not get the cups of tea so she might as well have the flowers.

I ring Imogen and say that I do not want to tire her. I know she can only make one journey from Wiltshire. I know that she wanted to visit her friends in London while staying with me, and I have been looking forward to her company, but it is only right that she be at her grandmother's funeral. I have to choose that.

My wonderful girl rings on Sunday morning and says she will do both. She will arrive tonight with Lizzie and go back on Wednesday evening ready for her Thursday meeting, and will drive up alone on the Friday, just for the day.

Monday I get a call from the funeral parlour. 'We've got your mum here, nice and safe.' I picture her having a cup of tea with them. Imogen is out visiting, so I try on again the black dresses which Linda has lent me. The weather is hotter every day, and anyway, I am not sure if they suit me.

On Tuesday, Imogen comes with me to visit Sylvia, who has only seen the baby once, visiting in Wiltshire with me. Before we go I call the funeral place and tell them that I am not sure that I will come to see my mother, as I am scared. 'Oh, that's a pity,' the woman says in her sweet voice. 'They've tried ever so hard for you, to made her look nice.'

Yesterday I bought the sheet music for one of the pieces to be played at the funeral. The organist had the others, but not this one, and it is the most important. We drop it in on our way to Sylvia.

Now it is Wednesday and Vanessa is coming to see me to arrange the last details of the service. Imogen takes Lizzie and they go off to look after Molly. Her school has broken up for the holidays, but Anna's has not yet.

Vanessa arrives and we walk to the funeral parlour together. She goes in first into the tiny Chapel, telling me afterwards that she did this to make sure that everything was all right. Mother has had her hair done, and it is all white and fluffed up. It has not been done by the hairdresser in the Home, not the one who was better than mine, but still as good it seems. If Mother is looking down on the scene, she would no doubt tell me to go to the hairdresser who does it for corpses, so that I can get myself a nice man.

Mother does not look like herself, and when I say this to Gordon later he says, 'well it is not the person, is it?' But I do not mean because she is not here, I mean that her mouth is nothing like her mouth. The funeral lady explains it is because of gravity and way it drags down the muscles of the mouth. Her mouth looks grim.

Vanessa tells me that she has written a prayer and she tells me to hold my mother's hand with one hand and hers with the other. Then she reads: 'We thank you for all you taught us, that life should be more expansive. We are sorry it was not so for you, but hope that on some other plain, it is now.' I ask to be left alone, so Vanessa looks for the last time on Mother. 'Hasn't she got lovely skin.' She says.

Alone I ask silently for whatever there was between us, whatever the pull or link, that she will release me from it now. We run from the place.

'That young girl,' says Vanessa, 'the one who showed us into the chapel, wasn't she good looking?' I have prepared us a nice quiche and salad lunch courtesy of Rafe. Vanessa does not want alcohol so I give a coffee while I make myself a strong gin and tonic. We discuss the ceremony on Friday.

'You only have two days,' I say.

'You have done most of the work for me', she says, and once more I am pleased with my writing and the ease with which I wrote the eulogy. Usually the minister gleans the information about a person who has died from their relatives and friends, and then has to write it up. We walk together, in the heat, along the long road to where Anna lives, for Vanessa to meet Molly, Imogen and Lizzie. I am wondering about the black dresses in this weather.

After the visit, Vanessa needs to be shown to the bus stop near Anna's rather than coming all the way back to my house. As we walk together down my daughter's road I can see a bus coming. Arms outstretched to attract the attention of the bus driver, Vanessa and I run towards the bus stop, our long Indian skirts flying behind us. Running and running, enjoying the outing and forgetting it is all about death. 'See you Friday,' she calls as the bus pulls away.
'What are you going to wear? I call at her, but it is too late.

That evening, Gordon calls about the arrangements. I tell him I do not know what to wear. Hayley calls, back from Florida, and says she can find nothing suitable which does not need dry cleaning. She will have to buy something new tomorrow. Then Imogen has to go and I say goodbye to baby Lizzie, knowing that my daughter will be coming on her own in just over a day's time.

Thursday, and it is an extra monthly creative writing meeting. It is our annual competition day, and I wear for the first time my lovely summer dress, bought in a sale when out and about with Sylvia.

Friday, I get up and put on my bathroom airing rack the washing done overnight, on Economy Seven. I do some hand washing. Then I go to see Mother for the last time. She has not moved from when I saw here. She is not saying that I am late, or why can't I stay a bit longer, but I keep expecting her to tell me off. When I held her hand on Wednesday with Vanessa, I noticed her hands were soft and floppy, where I had expected them to be rigid. It is still the same.

Her finger nails are mauve, is it nail vanish? I ask the funeral lady and she tells me it is just the way the fingers go. I feel her body, but I can't feel all the way down. The covering of the coffin makes it like a canoe, so that the body is totally unreachable from the waist down. I can't see her feet. I seem to be almost panicking and wonder if it is because I don't believe she is all there. Her poor twisted feet. 'Are her feet there?' I ask.

'Oh, yes,' says the woman, 'she is all there.' I kiss her forehead and then tuck the last card she received, the one from Hayley, into her hands. She has no rosary, no jewellery, and no other presents. The card shows a beautiful, old fashioned lady, in a long and lovely dress.

'You can come anytime,' says the sweet woman as I leave, 'any time you are passing. We always have the kettle on.'

She explains how some relatives want to do this, particularly in the case of an old person who has lost their partner of a lifetime. It is someone to talk to, someone to talk to about the deceased.

I think, as I walk home, what an intimate thing it is, this funeral arranging. Afterwards, you could well feel an emotional attachment to the funeral people, similar to that warmth you can have towards nurses, after an operation or the birth of your child, or those who have been close to you in a very private way. The funeral lady would be the last link with the dead, part of the bridging time. The in-between person to whom you went when it had only just happened, and so a link to when the person was alive, certainly to the time when their body was still here. Yes, arranging a funeral is an intimate business.

Back home, I have time to call the two Homes my mother was in, before her last eight days, which were spent in the Nursing Home. They had heard of her death and I talk to them about the hoist and my other experiences of Henley.
The Manager in Fawsett House says that he would 'go bananas,' if he saw any of his staff transporting clients like that, and both Homes are shocked that I was asked to arrange the removal of my mother's body, telling me that they always do that for relatives.

(Henley have still not found the corner unit.)

Anna rings and asks how 'Nanny is going to get there.' Well, I shouldn't think she is in any hurry, and I feel like saying, 'on the bus,' but know she means are we going to follow the hearse in our cars or not.

Imogen arrives an hour before the service. I wore an old T-shirt and thin skirt to the undertakers' so now I try on my friend's black dresses and something else. It is not black, but a plain navy blue dress that I bought with my hostess points at one of my clothes parties. It is not a summer dress, but is cooler than the others.

Between Imogen and me we decide on the navy dress and I put on my gold plated earrings, another free gift this time from a jewellery party. I am a walking advertisement for Hilary.

Imogen drives me and one by one the family arrive in the car park, my siblings, my children, their families, my friends. I hear Anna say to Gregory and Holly, 'now you know what is going to happen, don't you?' It is their first funeral. What a good mother she is. I see Elaine with her eldest brother, and with Albert's son. Victor and his wife are accompanied by her sister and brother-in-law, and I think, how kind of them to come. I see Carers from the home Mother left only a few weeks ago. Vanessa has been here for over an hour to check on everything, and joins us all now as we gather outside the chapel.

Most have gone inside now. Hayley comes up to me and gives me a tiny packet. In it is an angel, which she pins on my dress. We see the car coming slowly. Mother arrives grandly, at the end. Like the Queen of Sheba. Like a bride.

The car stops at a distance and a figure gets out. She is wearing a suit and a hat with a veil, and black gloves. She steps smartly towards us and I think, human beings do the very best they can. Wouldn't you say? She gives me the sheet music I bought. They have copied it, she says. I got my photographs back this morning when I went to see Mother. She asks that all but the chief mourners go inside and she will bring the car up slowly. She walks briskly away. Rafe stands by me, and looks into my face. He looks so loving, so concerned about me. Then he asks if he can hold the music for me during the service, and takes it from me just as my children all go in.

Everyone is now inside leaving my mother's four children alone, except for Vanessa. The car arrives and the back door is opened. 'Right, gentlemen', says the lady funeral director, and Mother is on their shoulders. Vanessa is in front of the coffin and we walk behind, walking in to the organ playing, 'We'll Gather

Lilacs in the Spring Again', which Mother sang in the war. I put those words on her flowers from me too. Just the idea that there might be a future. A time when we will do anything, and something nice, like picking flowers.

And maybe she will bring me tea on a saucer. Unspoiled. And I will not be scalded – have my sexual area hurt – as I have been. Only my inner cup of joy will run over.

Vanessa reads the eulogy which is mostly mine, but has additions from Valerie and Gordon, and then she reads a poem I wrote about my mother twenty years ago. We sing a hymn, because my sister wanted a hymn. Then Grace from Mother's Spiritualist Church gives an address – the one who was at Mother's ninetieth birthday party. She tells how my mother always liked to be called Mrs. and her surname. Well, I think, she would not have wanted to be called Nellie, would she? But no, it was the way with that generation. Even with mine for a long time. When I first had children, we mother's, although only in our twenties, called each other Mrs. Of course Vanessa calls Mother Eleanor throughout.

At the end, we all leave the chapel to the tune of the Beatles, 'Yesterday.' Outside one of the Carers is crying more than anybody else. She was my mother's Key Worker, who came with us to Tesco's. I am annoyed that two or three are carrying their floral tributes in their hands. They brought the sprays with them, rather than have then sent, so these go straight onto the ground with the ones brought from the coffin and the car. Mother never got them.

'We thought we'd just pick them up on the way,' one of the culprits say to me, 'you said you wanted flowers.'

'But I wanted them for her. I wanted the car to be covered. I wanted her massed with flowers.' But the woman just looks at me puzzled.

Vanessa comes with us to the reception, just briefly before dashing off to finish her Sunday sermon. 'Do you know where to get a bus? I ask her at the hotel. She does, she kept her eyes opened for bus stops as Imogen drove us to the hotel.

My daughter will need to leave early too, to get back to Wiltshire and her baby.

'Will you do my funeral? Sylvia asks Vanessa.

'We didn't know all that,' my sister's children say to me 'about Nanny we mean.' Did my mother only load me with her life?

My mother's cousin, Barbara, has come, the daughter of grandmother's artist brother Len. She asks me about my mother, about how difficult she was and why she was so unhappy. I tell her of the sexual abuse by Uncle Olly. Then she tells me that she was abused too, by the same uncle, and repeatedly, over a long period of time. I ask her if she ever told anyone and she says she didn't. She did not know that it wasn't normal, wasn't what happened to everyone. 'They were a strange family,' she tells me, as she has told me many times before.

'I didn't know she was called Eleanor,' says Elaine, joining us. 'Not until today, I always thought Nellie was her actual name.'

One of the two people in my life, who have refused to stop shortening my name, said something very similar to that. They stated that I was not christened Patricia. As so often happens, I was struck dumb, but inside I replied, 'no, I was not christened at all. But it is what my Birth Certificate says.'

Mother hated `Nellie.' What might it have been like had she been an Eleanor? Gregory says he thought the funeral was good. Rafe comments on the music. 'What was that music played when the coffin went? It is famous, the theme tune of more than one film.'

It is a lovely day and there were so many people for her.
Vanessa led the proceedings beautifully and nobody could have wished for a better funeral. Some old people only get a handful of mourners, my mother got over forty. It was a hot day, but I am not too hot in my dress, as I am usually cold anyway. A lovely day for her, and the best we could all do, other than the flowers that were dragged along like big carpet bags.

And she sank to the air of . Ever since the nurse said that of my mother's figure and I saw my mother as a sleeping beauty, there could be nothing else. The coffin stood to the right of the minister and, at the time of committal, Vanessa moved and stood close to

Mother, standing to attention with what looked to me like honour and love, as Mother slowly left us.

Awake unto – Me.

Chapter 36

The next day, Saturday.

After the funeral yesterday, Hayley and Gordon came home with me for an hour, but the rest of the evening stretched ahead, and now today stretches even longer. Why did nobody wonder how I would feel today, whether I had anything to do?

Gordon drove me home from the hotel, as Imogen had already left, and we talked about our mother before Hayley arrived. I said there was some growth, some move on towards the end. I told him how Mother said she would go in a plane now. How she said she had come to terms with why her mother had needed to go in the shop. 'I saw a move on too,' Gordon told me. 'You remember how she was always going on about wanting to see me with some nice girl? Well, only a month or two ago she said to me, 'perhaps you are better on your own'.'

Then Hayley came and I admired her new dress. She told me again that she arrived home from Florida and lay on the bed going through the possibilities of what to wear for the funeral and that in the end she decided she would have to go out and buy something new. 'I can't believe women,' said Gordon. He looked at me, 'I could not believe it last night when you said to me on the phone that you were worried about what to wear.'

*

Now, what can I do to get though the day? Most of my days are a getting though, a making do. I have ironed yesterday's washing, done a few more hand washing bits, cleaned a pair of shoes, then had a coffee and half a cigarette. I smoke five cigarettes a day, but in halves, so that I get ten goes. Meals, drinks, and half cigarettes break up the day. I run to the corner supermarket for something nice to eat for lunch. make a birthday card, and receive calls from each of the children asking me how I feel. I do not know how I feel about my mother. I say I am lonely and have nothing to do, nowhere to go, nobody to see. They all have arrangements, and engagements for today, but say that they care.

I break up time, fill it up. Why did I not make a space for Mother that last day? A walk to the library and back has used up an hour. I also photocopied the crossword from the Daily Telegraph. A murder mystery book and a crossword are as much a treat as my lunch. After lunch I make some cakes. I like a cake with my afternoon cup of tea and they are too expensive to buy. I make little cupcakes for myself, and flapjack for the family. Gordon ate the last of the flapjack yesterday.

What can I do before it is time for my evening meal? I could read, I think, as the long lonely afternoon and evening stretch out before me. I read for a while but am restless. I start the crossword, realising that I could have used Rafe's money to buy a newspaper, but either way I know I will end up checking the crossword in libraries, and I am so tired. I look again at the profile of the man in my introductions booklet. He says he is thirsty for knowledge. The only other person I have ever known to use the word 'thirsty' about their brain is me. I am always saying that I am thirsty for ideas. If I write to this man then I can go and post it, more exercise, more time used, but I am not sure. I could do some writing instead.

Maybe I will cut back my bushes myself.

My attitude to Circle Dancing is changing too. I have been a few times of late, and do not find it so boring. The music makes it peaceful. And meditative. And healing. Of course it does.

I am not allowing myself to think how awful my mother's end was. I feel as lonely and exhausted as ever, but as ever half hopeful –

Gasping to stay alive, in the hope that one day I will have a life.

Chapter 37

Something new comes into my musing. A final piece to the jigsaw I am trying to put together, another piece towards the whole picture of understanding. Victor has sent me a piece he has written about our mother. He did not have time to do it for the funeral, but thinks we night use it now, since Vanessa has suggested we hold a memorial service. Victor is older than I am, and writes of a time I do not remember much, when he was six and I just four.

He tells of the time we were evacuated in the war. Mother came too, because she had a baby, my sister. We went to Wales and his story says that we stayed here and there, as Mother tried to find somewhere suitable for us to live. At first she was placed in other families' homes, where the homeowner was there, and she was in constant clashes with them. She ended up in a cottage in the middle of nowhere. I can remember it myself a little.

My brother says that most of the time we had the place to ourselves but What I remember is that we shared it with another woman and her son. But at least the two women were on equal footing, and that I assumed was why Mother settled for it. There was no water except what she had to carry from a pump a hundred yards away, and he tells of Mother melting snow in saucepans to get us water when the pump froze, I remember that too. What I did not know was that the cottage had neither gas nor electricity. She had to cook on a wood fire. No electricity meant we had no radio, so what did she do in the evenings?

Before reading this account, I have never given much thought to how it must have been for our mother during that time in Wales. To be sharing a small place with another family. To be looking after two children and a baby with neither electricity nor running water. To have to walk far to a pump for water, and then have that freeze up in winter. Her loneliness without her beloved radio must have been great.

The other family was not there all the time that we were, so for some of the time Mother was without adult company. Perhaps the other woman might have been a cause of friction, for our mother did not get on with people. I have always felt she shunned other mothers for fear they would see her short comings. She had fled the first more comfortable homes because of the arguments which arose between her and the owners. I have often thought that her isolation came from a fear of censure, but maybe there were other reasons too. Childhood abuse, especially by a relative, can cause you to turn away from close intimacy, for you have learned that there is no one you can trust, another woman for company or not.

The daily grind of looking after three children, including a baby, in such circumstances would have been nothing but misery. And an extraordinary feat of endurance and duty since she did not particularly like children. A radio would have been the difference between heaven and hell. But she did not have that.

What shocks me most of all in my brother's account is his dismissal of our mother's suffering in that cottage in Wales, his brushing away the possibility that she may have been justified in feeling wretched, even in hitting out. For it was in that war time cottage that she held the knife to her little boy's throat.

He writes that in his opinion many people today might welcome the fun of roughing it like that as a 'different' holiday – some kind of 'yuppie' reversal roles of slumming it. He claims that she would not have adapted to the life as anybody else might because she was spoilt. She was a spoilt little girl and therefore three children with no water or electricity would be too hard for her where it would not have done others! Spoilt? She lived until her late twenties behind a shop. It had no bathroom, only an outside toilet and a kitchen sink.
The shop was in a slum street whose life depressed her. She spent the years between schooldays and marriage washing up for everyone else. Before being evacuated she had spent five years in war time London, looking after first one baby then three, with little money, no support, and no love. From babyhood she had grown up with a mother who had no time for her.

What infuriates me is the realisation pf the `spin` which has been written around my mother`s life. A reality created which enabled people to put her down. I do not blame my brother. Someone told him that our mother was spoilt. But who told him that? Was it his father? Mother's brothers?

The word 'spoilt' would have coloured all her complaints from then on. Any time she complained of being left all the working week while my father slept at the shop because of the late hours and early starts – all that to create a fortune for Grandmother and Albert, not a penny of the profits for us – only Dad`s lowly pay. All the time she lived on a shop Manager's salary, not enough to clothe her children let alone have much for herself, all the time she had a husband whose hours meant no social life. All the time her life was drudgery, poverty, and kids, and relatives who gave more criticism than help. All the time her own mother was crippled and could not contribute even the minimum of childcare as most grandmothers do. She would be neither listened too, nor helped, in any way.

There was nothing wrong with her life. She was just spoilt. What a clever way of silencing someone and keeping them where they are. What a clever way of diverting attention away from your own contribution to their life. The calling of my mother 'spoilt' makes me think how women have been described as hysterical. It reminds me how so often in our history we are sold the picture of the mad woman in the attic, the nagging wife, the woman who is neurotic and insane, while her suffering husband is a saint; and nobody looks to see what she is nagging about, or how less than a saint is the poor man.

*

` Now I see her face, The old woman abandoned, The moon her only companion.'

I read more of Basho`s poetry.

I think of my mother, on a seat in the high street, already out so early in the morning. (And often, out with my mother, trailing to pub from car park on a wet and blustery Sunday, I have seen us reflected in a shop window and thought, two old girls, both used by nature to produce four children, and then left to rot.)

But on that Surbiton seat at eight in the morning! What was she running from? In that frenzy which took her out of her bed and away from her flat, before any place of cheer was even open? What was she running from when she was found dying down by the Thames that day?

I wonder if it was from herself. Was she frightened of herself though she didn't know why? Driven to run from whatever drove her, and I think that something could have been anger. Anger at her womanhood, destroyed by experiencing sex for the first time too young, and not appropriately, for having her sex outraged by a weak and selfish male. Did she have to run from that anger, for fear of what it might make her do?

I hear that Trudi is in hospital, she who was abused by her father and who I thought had coped so well, so differently to my mother. But it gets you in the end, doesn't it?

Where does the blame lie for my mother's un-fulfilled life and her damage of me? And what of that damaging of me, her only ally? It is obvious to me now that if someone has no-one, and then they find one person, then they will be terrified of losing that only one. They would do all they could to disempower them, but would also keep proving to themselves, that they will never leave them, by constantly pushing to see how far they could go. 'If she has taken this, yet another abuse, then she will never leave me.'

So where does the blame for it all lie? Only this week I heard at my literature class a poem by W H Auden in which he says that families are the place where we go mad. So does the blame sit with Jack for working in a shop, too busy to notice the wicked uncle? Or does it lie with Mother's brothers for putting her down? With Albert in particular for landing her behind a shop, the life she had wanted to escape? With my father for getting pregnant a girl who had no desire for marriage, and for giving her three more children whom he could not afford to support?

What about Mother's great-grandfather who disinherited her side of his family, so denying her the lady's life she felt she was born to? A life which was perhaps in her bones? What about living through two world wars? The bomb which fell nearby, when she was a small child? The bombs which filled her with terror when she had small children of her own? There was her ill health too. Who was responsible for that? Society? Her husband? Her family? That scene of the asthma attack outside the holiday chalet haunts me – especially now. Had she always been gasping for breath, and in the end had no strength to gasp anymore?

There can be no blame, for if one damages another, then who first damaged him? Who knows where it all began, but the first pain set rolling a whole history of toppling dominoes. Maybe

Mother's mother would not have bought her shop if her father had not been cut off without a penny for marrying the wrong girl, but how can we set blame at the door of that Peircey household when such were the class mores of the time? If my uncle destroyed his sister's life because his mother emasculated him, Is it not understandable to create a world, a reality, which is more comfortable for you?

I cannot blame my father and now can only think of his life with sorrow. He worked a long week, long days, in a shop for a wage which gave us only a bare existence. Hard enough to do the hours he did, but he also had our mother constantly nagging him to change his job, nagging that he should never have let Albert get him into it. Apart from the fact that some of us children saw him simply as someone who was mean because he could not give us much, he had little time in which to get to know us. He always seemed to look angry, and what I can always picture in my head are his angry eyes. Surely that anger was really about himself, about his failure as a provider and his act of defence was to direct it at us. He had an unloving marriage and little cheer in his life. What if he did spend some money on records, or even on other women? I am glad that he found some kind of safety valve. I hope those treats gave him something to look forward to, and eased his pain. I imagine he was inwardly very alone.

If I were to place any blame at all, it would be on Henley, Mother's final Home, with its miserable food, its mean little cupboard of an office, its tea in a mug, no secretaries, no activities and some days no Manager. Never enough nurses to give time to transporting clients with dignity, but strung up on a hoist. Not enough staff to spare one to sit with her dying, and no one with the sensitivity, medical knowledge, the psychological insight or the training – whatever it needed – for someone to urge me to stay that day.

Maybe nobody can ever be blamed for anything. Most people do what they really think they are entitled to do, because of their psychology. Sometimes, I have been amazed at the way people justify themselves.

What does surprise and indeed distress me is that other people stand by and watch someone suffer or be ill-treated. Why does no one ever say, `what is happening to this person?` or ` why are we standing by while somebody is treated like that?`

Has nobody heard what Edmund Burke said? – `The only thing necessary for the triumph of evil, is for good men to do nothing.`

If, deep down, I knew she was probably dying, surely qualified nurses must have known it too? Oh, if only they had suggested it might be a good idea if I had stayed, `just in case,` or why not call me back in time, before it was too late?

Why did they let me go home? Why did I go? So here we come full circle and I failed my mother in the end. I went because my visit to her was part of a list, and I had to move on to the next item, to have a cup of tea, a cake and half a cigarette. Then I would work through the list, do some writing, call my daughter, and maybe flick through a magazine (passed on by a friend) for the pictures I could use to make my cards. Then it would be cook and eat my dinner, do my meditation, have a bath and finally read myself to sleep.

I made my life – not bearable – but I suppose hopeful, safe, or something by dividing it up like this. Maybe structures are to do with safety. It was all working to a purpose: exercise, meditation, writing – all a striving to earn a better life. Exercise to hang on to youth, meditation to reach a higher consciousness, sell a book to bring money, success, a better self-image. It was all in a way an outstretching of hands in prayer for a more fulfilling life in every way, and particularly for a lover. I was frenziedly gasping to stay alive in the hope that one day I would have a life. I have spent my whole life trying to get the things most people take for granted, have felt like I was crawling along on my hands and knees, gasping for breath. Just to get my basic needs met.

I would not have had to be doing this, Mother, if you had not disempowered me (sadly, I might have had more for you – money, the nice house with a granny flat, a helpful son-in law. I would have been there, forever the dutiful, the trying to please, bringing tea so carefully, not to spill it in the saucer. Probably it was only I who always knew you wanted a cup and saucer not a mug). But you would have lost control of me, wouldn't you, if I had had someone to champion me?

But if all who damaged Mother can be understood and forgiven, so must she. There is no blame for the frittering and gallivanting, the gadding around, those were her safety valves. There is no blame for the knife. Had she murdered my brother and paid with her life, what an indictment on a world that makes a young mother flee her home town and what family support she might have, putting her in a lonely cottage without water, electricity, gas – or a radio.

For the woman who left her children to make their own beans and bread (oh, beans and bread, the last meal I saw put in front of Mother) – the only escape, respite, was her radio and cup of tea. Possibly the mother with thirteen children who let the bad leg get so infected that it had to be amputated and then ignored that, had no respite at all.

There is no coping with hard times when there is no let up, no joy. In Primo Levi's 'If this is a man,' I find the words; `we who are half crazy with the dreary expectation of nothing'.

Maybe it is not the thought of death, or not only death, which depresses, but being denied the joys of this life while we still live, joys which, if we have them, make death a fair price. It is said that the greatest pleasure available to human beings is that of sex. It is possible that such experience might bring a bright light to other lacks and the man might bear the grinding job, and the woman the drudgery.

This joy which might put an end with the toppling dominoes is however available to few. For it seems to me that, although since the nineteen sixties we have been allowed 'to do it', to have sex, we do not usually know how.
Very rarely do people reach satisfaction. For if people had the joy which eases pain, why would they all be hurting each other so much? Why would the sexual scene be as it is, with men guilty of deviancy and sexual crimes? Where sex is considered to be for the young and beautiful so that men want younger women and women go into age unloved?

Surely it is immature, sexually, for a man to take a girl who is not interested, as my father did because of his own needs?
If the man is not giving pleasure to the woman, then the whole thing cannot really be satisfying to him, for the ultimate bliss comes from the intimacy of soul with soul. So many men cannot

satisfy their women because they will not attend to their women's needs or requests. The male ego will not let them be told, and they call the woman frigid.

When a man of note was reported to have been caught kerb crawling, a psychologist was questioned about this kind of behaviour on the radio, and he said that men are not capable of the close relationship needed for the marital bed, and so have to seek anonymous sex. Listening to him I thought, oh, that's all right then!

I once read a letter in a magazine's problem page where a wife complained that her husband insisted on wearing plastic baby pants as a sexual kick. The magazine Auntie replied that men have more fetishes than woman, and the woman should get some fetishes of her own! When a government minister was caught with his trousers down, a very well-known agony aunt said publicly that men have to go elsewhere because their wives, over time, lose interest in sex. I thought what a traitor to your own sex you are.

We accept this and so it remains the same. There is not the spiritual growth for the truly intimate relationship which brings life-long and increasingly joyful sex. Women do not lose interest, and if they appear to be frigid it is because they are disappointed. They become bitter and the bitterness causes them to treat their daughters in a way which will ensure that they have the same fate. The bitterness breeds those pursed-tight mouths you see on older women, with tiny lines around them like spokes.

I read that the deepest of chariot wheels in ancient Pompeii were those on the route to the brothel. Men go for ease elsewhere, to pornography, to strip clubs, to prostitutes. To little girls.

What I saw in the residents in mother's Retirement Home was the madness born of misery. The hell of facing imminent death after a lifetime of un-fulfilment is surely reason enough for creating new realities and appearing demented. I read that women who have had female circumcision can sometimes barely walk. To me that is a symbol that there is no going forward without sexual joy. No spiritual going forward. Could my mother's twisted feet be a symbol of her lack of spiritual moving forward, and was that a sign of her own brand of female circumcision? Did childhood sexual abuse programme her for a sexless life? Was the blocking out of her ability to experience sex to the full affected by her childhood sexual abuse?

It is said that to be sexually abused by a father teaches you that nobody can be trusted. You have been betrayed by the first and most important man in your life, therefore you see all men as abusers. And so they often are, of course they are. And you would have trusted an uncle too, wouldn't you?

I have heard depression called lack of self-esteem. What I see in my mother and women like her is the ignominy of being no-one's darling. To most, childbirth is pain beyond belief, and to some it is an embarrassing, even humiliating activity.
Together with abortions and some forms of contraception and drudgery, we suffer the rough end of womanhood. To balance that we need what is not always there, the best end of being female, being seen to be other than the apron. To be cherished. Well served in bed. To be lavishly provided for, and a bejewelled darling.

Nobody speaks with the tongues of angels at all – not even as sounding brass or tinkling cymbals – rather they can scarcely talk at all if they do not have love. Consider my mother's faint writing, the fading voice and the handwriting which was illegible all her life. Messages scrambled like letters in bottles thrown out to sea with little hope. That resigned look that came from abuse which was not made right by some healing love.

All of us are damaged, yet not all of us reach redemption. When I think of those who abuse because they were so badly treated, I wonder why they don't sometimes step aside and ask themselves what they are doing and why, and do they really want to hurt this person? Does it really ease their pain?

And is the greatest holocaust this Rumpelstiltskin thing? All the evils of society and individuals which work towards a mother not being able to love her child. The mother who left her baby in its bath. The mother who rejected the little girl who brought the tea cup on a saucer, forever, like an offering. The mother who held a knife at her little boy's throat Money, abuse, whatever is those mothers' reasons, it is her loss not that of the child. He may be able to make it on his own, in some way. But hat life should spoil, for mothers, the golden child.

Mother stepped outside, at least once to my knowledge. Until Gordon was about two, our parents lived with four children in a tiny rented flat in Leytonstone, a mile or so from Grandmother's shop. They had long been on the list for council housing and had waited in vain. Then Mother's mother offered to buy us a house. The only house my father could find, in between his shop hours, was in Essex.

At the last minute a council house was offered to us, and it would have been near the old shop, near her mum, but my mother rejected it. It turned out that she hated the village in Essex where we went, but even before knowing that, she wouldn't have wanted to leave her mother and her aunties.
But she rejected the council place because it would have meant us going to a rough school, and so she is redeemed.

And coats on our beds instead of blankets? Was that neglect, or care? She did her best to keep us warm.

All my spiritual teachings have been that sex is good, that it is essential for inner health. Gill Edwards in 'Living Magically' says that we cannot become spiritual if our needs are not met, and in his famous triangle, Abraham Maslow puts sexual fulfilment very high on his list of needs. I read so much that points to the fact that it is only through sexual ecstasy, that we reach a higher spiritual state.

It is interesting that some religions drive sex underground. They make it, if not sinful, then base. The resulting frustration and denial means that it can find room only in sordid practice.
One philosopher says that you will not change the world until you change the heart of man. So if sexual fulfilment will raise us to a higher state – to our kingdom of heaven – is there in fact something sinister in the establishment, including the church, making it outlawed?

Man has been encouraged to seek other pleasures and fulfilments – side-tracked you might say, with material gain and cerebral exercise. How interesting that humbler joys are given a sexual description, music is orgasmic, so also can be mathematics; and the stroking a cat or even a violin can be spoken of with sensual delight. Vicarious satisfaction. Making do. For if this veto – this climate of opinion and dictate – were withdrawn might not the state of man be nearer to that of angels?

And might not then the ordinary man become a threat to what is the status quo?

For what people fear most is to them far worse that all the ills our unhealed state creates, all the many kinds of wars both large and small. (Why, even natural disasters are attributed by some thinkers to the inner state of man). But what is most feared is change. For, while change may be for the better, it may not. For the disadvantaged it is more likely to be beneficial than for those more favoured. And it is with the latter that the power lies. They are stronger and their collective consciousness rules the world.

So change is avoided and anything that might promote it; any activity which brings enlightenment and advance. The potential empowerment wrought by sexual fulfilment is made unlikely, through the debasing of sex. And awareness brought about by intellectual growth is quashed by the `divide and rule` ethos I believe to be behind the demise of Adult Education. The same aim which is behind the encouragement of people to work – alone – at home.

Oh, my business which did not survive because of the economic and other forces around at the time. How I wanted to create groups where people would grow. And, to quote the words above the stage of Richmond Theatre: `to wake the soul by tender strokes of art.`

I want to do my part, in the greater story. Like Louis Macneice in his Autumn Journals, I do not want to turn my face to the wall, but rather let 'my feet follow my wider glance.'
I can only try, through my meditation and my walks with angels – and my spiritual books. And it was Mother gave me the first one of those books, wasn't it?

*

Most of the family has Mother's thick hair and in this child or that grandchild I spot the auburn lights. I have her good skin and very blue eyes. Some of us use her words, `dinky`and `nobby' for small or handy things, and 'oo-er`! My son still calls me 'ducks.'

It was only after she died that I realised how she used to carry her bag. You know in those early days, how you keep thinking you are seeing your mum? You see an older lady with white fluffy hair, a blue dress, and a cardigan, and a handbag, held straight down. We carry ours over our shoulder, or clutched up to our boobs with bent arm. They hold their short handled bags with their arms straight. I saw a woman and thought it was her and noticed the bag and remembered. I looked at my photos and there she was at thirty, at sixty, at seventy and beyond, carrying it in exactly the same way.

I look as a scene flickers on my memory screen. There is the whole family, and my sister and I have handbags like Mum`s. We got them new for Christmas and we are taking them out for the very first time. There we are, at least for a moment, being a family and going to a pantomime, as we often did on Boxing Day. And I think to myself, they did their best, our parents, didn't they?

I see the rose that blew off my father's coffin to land at Mother's feet. So my little icing sugar dad – oh, he made and decorated wedding cakes, didn't he? My little bridegroom dad, did bow to his bride. In the end.

The Last Visit

They told me that Mother was not well as soon as I arrived at the Home that Sunday, and they had sent for a doctor.
They showed me to her room. She was alone in her little bed and looked grey and hollow cheeked. She did not have the white fluffy hair washed and set by the hairdresser who is better than mine. Her hair was dark grey, flat and greasy.

I know that she was hard work for them in the last few weeks at Churchfield House, with her not eating and hitting out at them. She had been at this last Home for over a week and she was moved here because nurses are equipped to deal with the less physically able. They might have at least washed her hair. Or asked me to. I did not take in its state until this last day.

As I walked up to the bed in her room, I was met with a sort of rasping groan coming from her. 'What?' I sat on the bed. I listened to the rasping and guessed she was saying. 'Go home?' I asked. She nodded.

I wanted to play the tape, but they had lost it again. I sat next to her on the bed and began to stroke her. If only I could mediate and play that tape at the same time, I thought, that might bring her to the serenity I so wanted for her. I started to meditate, hoping that my raised unconsciousness would raise hers, that the higher consciousness I was reaching for would somehow touch her too. I mediated and stroked her at the same time.

'Leave me alone,' she slowly moaned, so I stopped and did not know what to do. Then I leaned over her and stared into her eyes. I smiled with my mouth and my eyes, and she smiled at me with her lips and her eyes. It seemed to me that she looked surprised, happy, even excited.

I tell her that I am going to write a book about her awful life. I can see that she hears.

Her tongue was coated in bright white, thick and cracked. hunted for the tape with Esme; we were looking in a store room directly opposite Mother's bedroom with both doors open, so that she could see us. She seemed to be looking at us from a distance which was not just physical. It seemed she was looking as us, as if to say, what are they messing about at? I felt as if we two were in the busy life, while she was in another, one where you can think of nothing but how ill you feel. We were apart.

My statutory visiting time was finishing. I was going home to a cup of tea and homemade cake and half a cigarette stood in the doorway and blew a kiss towards my mother in her bed, thinking, `I wonder if I will ever see you again`. And went.

How long did she lie alone? Was it from my visit, ending at three to that of the doctor, at four, then to the administration of medication, and the blackmail trip to the toilet? How soon after the doctor's call would they have got her the required medication? I hope that the time was broken up more than that, the long-time from when I left until they 'looked in on her' at seven-thirty, just ten minutes before she died.

Did she lie there between those visitations looking resigned as when I saw her on the hoist, as when I saw my dad bashing her back? Did she lie there feeling miserable and lonely, physically suffering, as when she sat outside the holiday chalet having an asthma attack?

Well, Dad, Mum did die, and it was my fault. My fault that she died alone

The Regulator of Nursing Homes with whom I have been

corresponding about the way Henley is run has told me that some people die quickly, but she looked ill when I left at three and did not die until twenty to eight. When I telephoned Esme at seven, I was told that she was a lot better. All the time, during the telephone conversation between seven and seven twenty, did she start to die then? Was she feeling very ill, feeling lonely, feeling scared? Feeling resigned?

Did they look in on her at seven thirty, or was it just before calling me at ten to eight? Did they look in after she had died? I left her groaning and moaning. Did she moan for the rest of the time, right to the end?

*

Did she rasp to go home, right to the very end?

Back before the lonely time with children.
Before the cottage with no radio.
Before the bashed back.
Before the bomb-filled London with babies.
Before that other bomb when she was a baby herself.
Before the putting down by brothers.
Before the spiteful nuns.
Before the broken arm and the curse,
And the cosy uncle who betrayed her trust,
Before whatever happened on those dark stairs.
Back with Mum at the very beginning,
The time when she might still have been all right.

Beautiful Dreamer

Epilogue

What was wrong with Mother? Was I right to think of her as a sleeping beauty?

This is my conclusion, and I blame it on our culture, and the way that sexuality is not on the pedestal, but a virgin mother is. Without sexual fulfilment we have a stumbling block. We are not spiritual and are instead governed by the pleasures sent to distract us. We do not grow, and so we do not heal the world. I believe it is in our collective consciousness to keep the status quo because of the fear of change. So, we keep the money where it is, the power where it is, and the women where they are.

Mad, sad, or bad, with increasing age people become depressed. In fact they are in despair, because they have been cheated of all real joy.

Mother's last Nursing Home would have made anyone's end wretched, and the ethos at Henley is the ethos of our world. The place epitomises our capitalist culture where everything is run for the benefit of the shareholder or the tax payer, and not for the supplier, the employee, or the client.
All those years ago, in is play The Apple Cart, George Bernard Shaw named 'Big Businesses' as the chief evil.

Deepak Chopra, a spiritual teacher and medical doctor, disclaimed the common belief that man and woman, once one body, accidentally became divided, and that the sex drive is to do with us wanting to get back to that oneness again. Instead, he claims that we were purposely split so that we would seek oneness through sex; because only through sexual ecstasy will we reach our soul's fulfilment.

The consciousness which is going to be most strong in the collective one. It will be the consciousness of the successful, those who have the power because of money status or gender. The powerful ones who want the status quo, and spiritual growth in the masses would threaten it. So we are led to have their aims and values. The result is the various forms of theft – of exploitation – and the need to put women down in men whose male supremacy must not be threatened. To keep any disadvantaged, by race or anything else, where they are. In fear that change for some good might bring change for bad too.

If we were allowed to think instead of seeking worldly success, this might upset the apple cart.

For me this is what is behind the demise of Adult Education, the divide and rule, and why we are given as our 'gods' the rich and famous. Perhaps this is why, even on benefit, the State's calculations of our needs include a television. We watch the lives and problems and inner workings of soap characters, instead of dealing with our own.

We do not reach that spiritual stature which would bring realisation, that to hurt because we are hurt does not wipe out that hurt, and indeed erases any complaint we have, for we do no better than our destroyers!

The Vision

A few weeks before, I had a dream – was it a dream, or real? In some ways, perhaps we were on a different loop of time, or maybe it was something to do with astral bodies and parallel universes? Some scientists and philosophers do not believe that there is such a thing as time, or rather say that all `time` exists at the same time. And there are such things as parallel realities, aren't there?

I don't understand it, but I do know that some think there is more to our existence than ordinary people believe. Maybe when people are between this life and the next they see things differently, or have a different view of reality. Perhaps it was like the fantasy I had of my 'real' mother leaving her body when sitting in her dismal lonely lodgings in Worthing, and running off to the pier to dance, a beautiful lady in a lovely dress.

I would like to believe that the dream I had was somehow true for her.

Did I dream what would be real for her? Did she experience what I had dreamed, and wished for? All time exists at the same time, isn't that what the poets say? My favourite poet, T. S. Eliot wrote: 'Time present and time past are both perhaps present in time future.'

I dreamt that I was lying on her bed with my face, on her pillow, next to her face. And I knew that she was dying. We were in her little home bed, and I was lying on it with her.

We were just looking into each other's faces, all the time.

Beautiful Dreamer

www.ingramcontent.com/pod-product-compliance
Lightning Source LLC
Chambersburg PA
CBHW020747160426
43192CB00006B/266